I0817941

Praise for REWIRED

"The state of our nervous system shapes how we lead, how we work, and how we show up for ourselves and others. REWIRED *is an essential and empowering guide to building the calm, clarity, and resilience we all need."*

— **Arianna Huffington**, founder & CEO, Thrive Global

"Tapping has always been my gateway to slowing down, calming my mind, and getting fully present. I relied on it throughout my 12-year MLB career, long before I understood why it worked. Thanks to the evidence the Ortners lay out in this incredible book, I now know the feeling I had was real, neurological, and spot-on. Tapping truly unlocks so much. This book is an absolute must-read."

— **Sean Casey**, three-time MLB All-Star

"I've used Tapping for years. It's one of my favorite ways to reset and refocus fast. Your brain and body are always in conversation. REWIRED *shows how Tapping can reprogram that dialogue, quieting stress, sharpening focus, and freeing your best self to perform. It's not just self-care. It's neural training for modern life."*

— **Jim Kwik**, leading brain coach and *New York Times* best-selling author of *Limitless*

"REWIRED *breaks down the science of Tapping in a way that actually makes sense—and shows you exactly how to change the thoughts and patterns that keep holding you back. If you want emotional strength and real results, start here."*

— **Marie Forleo**, #1 *New York Times* best-selling author of *Everything Is Figureoutable*

"REWIRED *brings together solid science, relatable stories, and practical tapping sequences that clinicians and clients alike can put to work immediately. This is a powerful resource for real nervous-system transformation that anyone can use to genuinely transform their lives. It is an empowering roadmap for anyone ready to shift out of old patterns and into resilience."*

— **Professor Peta Stapleton**, author of *The Science Behind Tapping*

*"*REWIRED *is a clear, science-informed, and deeply practical road map for using Tapping to reshape the nervous system's habitual responses to stress in everyday life while opening the door to greater calm, confidence, and success. With a warm, conversational style, the Ortners blend research, real-world stories, and simple step-by-step practices so readers can actually 'recognize, interrupt, and rewire' not only the patterns that keep them stuck, but also the ones that are ready to grow into new strengths. It reads less like a clinical manual and more like a wise, good-humored guide at your side, making it a vital contribution to the Tapping field and a hopeful vision of what life can feel like when your nervous system is rewired for greater ease, resilience, and joy."*

— **David Feinstein, PhD**, co-author, *Tapping and The Energies of Love*

"The Ortner siblings' new book, REWIRED, *is a comprehensive guide to using the technique of EFT Tapping to transform your life. Written in an accessible conversational style, it includes sections on Tapping Scripts, Pop-outs, Case Examples (including his own), and Core Insights at the end of each chapter. The Ortners are able to interweave the science behind EFT and the proof of its effectiveness in a way that will go down easy for the layman, yet with enough footnotes and citations for the science-minded. Complex psychological problems are skillfully untangled one layer at a time. I wish this book had been available before I retired—my patients would have loved it!"*

— **Erik Leskowitz**, retired Harvard Medical School–affiliated psychiatrist

REWIRED

Also by Nick Ortner

The Tapping Solution

The Tapping Solution for Manifesting Your Greatest Self

The Tapping Solution for Pain Relief

The Tapping Solution for Parents, Children & Teenagers

The Big Book of Hugs: A Barkley the Bear Story

My Magic Breath: Finding Calm Through Mindful Breathing

Also by Jessica Ortner

The Tapping Solution to Create Lasting Change

The Tapping Solution's Daily Guidance Deck

The Tapping Solution's Kids Confidence: Affirmation and Tapping Card Deck

The Tapping Solution for Weight Loss & Body Confidence

Also by Alex Ortner

The Tapping Solution Planner

Gorilla Thumps & Bear Hugs: A Tapping Solution Children's Story

All of the above are available at your local bookstore, or may be ordered by visiting:

Hay House USA: www.hayhouse.com®
Hay House Australia: www.hayhouse.com.au
Hay House UK: www.hayhouse.co.uk
Hay House India: www.hayhouse.co.in

❁ ❁ ❁

REWIRED

The Breakthrough Tapping Method to Stop Overthinking, Calm Your Body, and Finally Feel at Ease

Nick Ortner,
Jessica Ortner,
and Alex Ortner

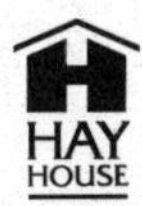

HAY HOUSE LLC
Carlsbad, California • New York City
London • Sydney • New Delhi

Published in the United States by: Hay House LLC, www.hayhouse.com®
P.O. Box 5100, Carlsbad, CA, 92018-5100

Cover design: Julie Rosenberger
Interior design: Julie Davison
Interior illustration: Courtesy of The Tapping Solution
Indexer: J S Editorial, LLC

Hardcover ISBN: 979-8-3186-0259-7
E-book ISBN: 979-8-3186-0260-3
Audiobook ISBN: 979-8-3186-0261-0

10 9 8 7 6 5 4 3 2 1

Printed in the United States of America

This product uses responsibly sourced papers, including recycled materials and materials from other controlled sources.

The authorized representative in the EU for product safety and compliance is Penguin Random House Ireland, Morrison Chambers, 32 Nassau Street, Dublin D02 YH68, Ireland. https://eu-contact.penguin.ie

To Mom & Dad,
whose love nurtured us
and courage inspired us

CONTENTS

Foreword

For more than 40 years, I've been obsessed with one question: What truly creates lasting change?

I'm not interested in hyped up, quick fixes. I'm interested in transformation that sticks. Transformation that rewires your nervous system, reshapes your emotional patterns, and frees you to become who you're meant to be.

That mission has taken me deep into human behavior, neuroscience, psychology, physiology, and energy medicine; anything that could help people break free from fear, pain, or limitation and step into a life they love. Along the way, I've seen tools that work for a moment . . . and I've seen tools that reshape people for a lifetime.

That's why I'm so passionate about this book and about what my partner Nick Ortner and his family are doing with EFT Tapping—a true tool for a lifetime.

I first met Nick not on a stage, but in the aftermath of a tragedy. When the Sandy Hook school shooting happened in his hometown, he and his siblings, Alex and Jessica, were already on the ground helping those impacted with Tapping. I came in to support, and what struck me wasn't just their compassion, but their quiet, steady leadership and commitment to helping those in need. Years before, Nick, Alex, and Jessica had been at my events as students, hungry to learn and to change their own lives. Now here they were, serving their community with a tool that was changing the lives of others in real time. These three have taken what started as curiosity and turned it into a movement that's touched millions of lives, and now they're giving you the exact method to transform yours.

At the core of this book is a technique called Tapping, which on the surface sounds deceptively simple: You use your fingertips to tap on specific points on your body while focusing on what's bothering you. But don't let the simplicity fool you. The roots of Tapping reach back thousands of years to the wisdom of acupuncture, an approach so enduring that its core principles are still used in hospitals around the world today to ease pain and promote healing. What's remarkable is how modern neuroscience now validates what those ancient healers understood intuitively: that stimulating specific points on the body can regulate the brain's stress circuits, calm the nervous system, and create real, measurable change.

Today, Tapping is one of the most researched interventions in emotional wellness, with over 300 studies documenting its effectiveness. Tests show it reduces cortisol levels. fMRI scans show it calms the brain. Gene expression research shows it creates change at the cellular level.

And the real-world results? They're remarkable. The Tapping Solution App has delivered over 32 million sessions, and the feedback is consistent: People feel significantly better after just one session. Take the Releasing Anxiety Tapping meditation, for example, which alone has been played over 1.7 million times. Users report an average reduction in anxiety of 40 percent in just nine minutes. Nine minutes. Not nine weeks. Not nine months. Nine minutes to measurably shift your nervous system. These aren't small numbers. These are millions of real people, getting life-changing results with something so simple and accessible that you can start today—right now—and feel the difference just a few pages into this book.

Over the years, I've seen Tapping calm schoolchildren who had witnessed horror, help first responders carrying unbearable weight, and bring relief to veterans haunted by PTSD. I've watched as the Ortners worked with people and shoulders dropped, breath returned, and hope came back to life . . . sometimes for the first time in years. I'm so proud of the work we've done together to bring Tapping to communities who need it most and to help more people access this powerful tool.

I don't just endorse this work from the sidelines. I use it myself. I've tapped before massive events. I've tapped in my personal life. I've tapped when I needed to shift my state fast. It's part of my own tool kit, right alongside the methods I've taught for decades.

That's why, when the Ortners launched The Tapping Solution App, I didn't hesitate to become their only outside investor and to record my own Tapping meditations for the app. Not just as a business decision (in fact I donate my percentage of sales to Feeding America and the Ortners match that percentage as well), but because I believe this work is needed now more than ever.

Which brings me to this book, *REWIRED*. This book couldn't be arriving at a more important time. We are living in one of the most stressful times in human history. Rates of anxiety, trauma, and burnout are skyrocketing. Our nervous systems are on overload from constant digital noise, global uncertainty, and personal pressures that never seem to let up. The old ways of coping simply aren't enough anymore. We need tools that don't just soothe for a moment, but that shift us at the deepest level.

And that's exactly what you're holding in your hands.

In *REWIRED*, Nick, Alex, and Jessica bring together years of experience, powerful stories, and the latest science on stress, trauma, and nervous system regulation. We've known Tapping works because we've felt it. Now we have the research and language to understand the transformations on a deeper level than ever before. But beyond that, this powerful book gives you the exact road map to use this technique for yourself. This isn't just theory. It isn't just about releasing stress. This book is about breaking free from your blocks, designing a life you love, and stepping into your fullest potential.

If you've ever wondered whether transformation is possible for you, hear me now: It is. I've lived it. I've witnessed it. The science is clear. The only question is: Are you ready to try it?

Don't just read this book. Do it. Tap along. Let yourself feel the shifts. Make the commitment right now that you're going to give this a real shot. Because when you do, you'll discover that freedom, peace, and power aren't out there somewhere . . . they've been inside you all along, waiting to be tapped into.

The time is now. The tool is here. The power is in your hands.

— Tony Robbins

Introduction

You Don't Have to Be Who You've Always Been

Let me ask you something.

When was the last time you did that thing? You know, the one you swore you'd never do again?

Maybe it was lying awake at 3 A.M., mind racing with worries you can't control. Maybe it was snapping at your kids when you promised yourself you'd be more patient. Maybe it was avoiding that opportunity because the fear felt bigger than the potential reward. Or feeling nothing when you desperately wanted to feel something, anything.

Whatever your "thing" is, I'm guessing it happened more recently than you'd like to admit.

And I'm guessing you've asked yourself the same question we all ask: *Why do I keep doing this? Why do I keep feeling this way?*

Here's what I know for sure: You're not broken. You're not weak. You're not destined to repeat these patterns forever.

You're just wired a certain way. And wiring can be changed.

The Promise of This Book

I'm going to make you a bold promise, and I want you to really hear it:

You don't have to be who you've always been.

You don't have to feel how you've always felt.

You don't have to do what you've always done.

That racing mind that keeps you up at night? It can quiet down. That anxiety that hijacks your body before presentations? You can release it. That numbness that makes you feel like you're watching life through frosted glass? It can thaw. That fear that's kept you small for years? You can outgrow it.

I know these sound like impossible claims. I know because I've watched thousands of people's faces when they first hear what Tapping can do. The skepticism. The "yeah, right" eye roll. The "I've tried everything and nothing works" exhaustion.

But here's what gets me up every morning, what has me jumping out of bed excited to share this work:

It's *true*. It actually works. And it works fast.

The Woman Who Changed Everything in 10 Minutes

Let me tell you about a woman at an airport. She's standing at the gate with her family, ready to board a flight to London. But she's sobbing. Her husband and children are huddled together, crying too.

She has a lifelong fear of flying. She thought she could do it and wanted desperately to do it, but now, faced with the plane, she can't. She's telling her family to go without her. To leave her behind.

A stranger watches from afar, her heart breaking for the family as she sees their tears and their struggle. She musters up her courage and approaches the family, asking if she can help. In the middle of the busy airport, with passengers streaming past, she pulls out her phone so they can listen to my guided "Fear of Flying" Tapping meditation together. They huddle together to hear the phone, the stranger guiding the woman through the Tapping process. Announcements are blaring in the background, the gate agents are sending last calls . . .

Ten minutes is all it takes. They finish tapping, and the woman looks up and says, "I think I can do this."

The once-terrified woman boards the plane first. She gives the kind stranger a thumbs-up as she passes in the aisle. Everyone goes to London, and no one is left behind.

Now, if you're wondering what exactly this "Tapping" thing is that they did, it's a simple technique where you literally tap with your fingertips on specific points on your face and body while focusing on what's bothering you.

These points are called acupressure points and were identified by traditional Chinese medicine thousands of years ago as key locations along the body's meridian system. Nowadays, modern science understands that they correspond to areas of the body rich in nerve endings, connective tissue, and microvascular networks that help send calming signals to the brain.

In simple terms, Tapping helps your body tell your brain, "We're safe now." This signal shifts your nervous system out of "fight-or-flight" mode and back into balance. Over time, it helps break the old stress patterns that keep you anxious, tense, or stuck.

We'll get into exactly how it works soon, but for now just know that this strange-sounding technique has been validated by over 300 peer-reviewed studies and has helped millions of people worldwide.

Think about it for a moment: If a stranger can help someone release their fear enough to get on a plane and have a once-in-a-lifetime experience, what could you do for yourself with this book in your hands?

What dreams could you finally chase? What experiences could you finally say yes to? And what feelings (freedom, joy, connection) are waiting for you on the other side?

Who You Are (And Why You Picked Up This Book)

You might be the successful professional who has it all together on the outside but lies awake at night with thoughts that won't shut off.

You might be the devoted parent who loves your kids fiercely but finds yourself repeating the exact patterns you swore you'd never pass on.

You might be the person who's tried everything—therapy, meditation, medication, self-help books—and still feels stuck in the same loops.

Or maybe you're someone who's mostly okay but knows there's something more. Some pattern, some limitation, some way of being that doesn't serve you anymore.

Here's what I know about you, regardless of which description fits: You picked up this book because some part of you believes change is possible. Even if it's just a tiny spark of hope buried under layers of disappointment and skepticism. Even if you've been let down before. Even if you're not sure you have the energy to try again.

That spark is all we need.

The Life You're Living vs. The Life That's Waiting

Before we go any further, let's get brutally honest about the life most of us are quietly living. A life where our minds race but our motivation stalls. Where our bodies feel more like a source of pain than a source of power. Where we feel either too much, getting hijacked by our emotions, or nothing at all.

We wake up tired. We push through our days on caffeine and willpower. We collapse into bed with our phones, scrolling mindlessly because we're too wired to sleep but too exhausted to do anything meaningful. We repeat this cycle day after day. Part of us is resigned to thinking this is just how life is, and another part of us has moments of hope that things will change one day. But they never do.

We've accepted this state as normal. We call it "adulting," "the daily grind," or just "life." We go about our daily lives and conclude that this low-grade misery is just part of being human.

But I'm here to tell you something that might sound radical: **Common is not the same as necessary.**

Just because everyone you know is exhausted, stressed, and running on fumes doesn't mean that you have to. Just because your co-workers joke about needing to distract themselves by scrolling through memes just to get through Tuesday doesn't mean emotional regulation is impossible. Just because your family has "always been anxious" doesn't mean you're doomed to pass that legacy on.

The REWIRED process is about moving you from the life you've accepted to the life that is actually waiting for you.

And let me tell you, our lives can be magical if we allow them to be so.

This isn't about a few small improvements. This is about a fundamental upgrade to your entire experience of being human.

The Great Forgetting

Most of us don't realize how far off track we are from a *good* and *magical* life.

In fact, we are like the proverbial frog in the pot of water. The temperature of our stress, our anxiety, our overwhelm has been turned up so gradually—an extra demand at work, another sleepless night, a new worry to carry—that we haven't noticed we're slowly being boiled in a broth of our own unease. We've simply adjusted to the rising heat.

Actually, scratch that. I've been using that frog metaphor for years, and it turns out I owe frogs an apology. I just learned that real frogs are smarter than we thought, and they actually hop right out when the water gets too hot.

Which means frogs have better boundaries than most of us.

We're the ones who stay in the pot, telling ourselves, "This is fine," while the bubbles start forming around us. We're the ones who've just gotten really, really good at convincing ourselves that slowly boiling is normal.

This new, simmering normal has its own set of unwritten rules that we live by without question:

It's accepting that a "good day" is simply one where you just managed to keep all the plates spinning, without any of them crashing to the floor.

It's believing that relentless exhaustion is the price of admission for being a responsible adult, and that having real energy is a luxury for the young or the unburdened.

It's a life where you spend more time managing your fears than you do chasing your dreams. Where you make decisions based not on what would light you up, but on what feels safest and least likely to end in failure or embarrassment.

Somewhere along the way, many of us went through a Great Forgetting. We forgot what it feels like to wake up feeling genuinely rested. We forgot what it's like to move through the day with a quiet mind, able to focus on one thing at a time. We forgot how to sit with the people we love and be fully *there*—not a million miles away, replaying a conversation or pre-planning tomorrow's to-do list.

We've forgotten that feeling at home and peaceful in our own skin is not a special occasion but our natural, biological birthright.

Or maybe, we never experienced any of that in the first place.

Either way, the dimmed-down state most of us walk around in has become so common that we think it's the *only* option. But there is another way to live. And that way is a heck of a lot better.

The Thread That Connects Every Struggle

In this book, we're going to explore the most common human struggles, the ones that millions of us face every single day:

- The mind that won't shut up at 3 A.M.
- The numbness that steals your joy
- The fears that steal your freedom

- The past that won't stay in the past
- The motivation that won't show up
- The exhaustion that sleep doesn't fix
- The body that feels like an enemy
- The relationships that replay the same painful dynamics

You might recognize yourself in many of these. Or all. Or just a few.

You might see your partner, your parent, or your best friend in some of them.

And here's the profound truth that changes everything:

Every single one of these experiences shares the same thread: You've been wired to respond this way.

Some of it's genetic. Some comes from experiences, especially early ones. Some developed as protection that you no longer need. But regardless of how the wiring got installed, it's all changeable through the same process.

That process is called Tapping, and it's going to rewire your default responses to life.

The Crossroads

Right now, as you're reading this, you're at a crossroads. Not the kind where someone lectures you about making the "right" choice, but the kind where you get to decide what happens next.

So let me ask you some questions:

- Do you like feeling this way?
- Is this who you want to be?
- Are you ready to stop being ruled by patterns you didn't choose?

If you answered yes to the first two questions, then you can close this book now. If you are 100 percent happy with how you feel on a daily basis, with who you are . . . I'm truly, truly happy for you. And you probably won't need this book. Maybe pass it to someone who's struggling.

Because change happens only when we want something different.

But if you're tired of being who you've always been . . . if you're ready to stop doing what you've always done . . . if you're willing to believe that your wiring can be updated . . .

Then let me show you what's waiting on the other side.

The Freedom Waiting for You on the Other Side

The point of this book, the entire reason I'm so fired up to share this with you, is to guide you out of Survival Mode and into a Rewired Life. A life where your default setting is not anxiety but peace. Not exhaustion but vitality. Not limitation but possibility.

By the end of this journey, you'll be well on your way to what I call the **7 Freedoms of a Rewired Life**.

The 7 Freedoms of a Rewired Life

1. **The ability to experience emotional freedom**—emotions flow through you instead of taking you down. You can feel without drowning and think without spiraling
2. **The ability to respond rather than react**—space between trigger and response, choice where there was only reflex
3. **The ability to feel calm in situations that used to throw you**—not fake Zen, actual nervous system regulation
4. **The ability to access energy you didn't know you had**—your cellular power plants working properly again
5. **The ability to feel at home in your body**—physical ease as normal, not exceptional
6. **The ability to trust yourself to handle whatever comes**—uncertainty becomes interesting, not terrifying
7. **The ability to show up as your *real* self**—instead of who you've always been or who you think you *should* be

What This Actually Looks Like in Real Life

Let me paint you a picture of what these freedoms mean in the mundane, beautiful reality of everyday life:

Your relationships transform because you're no longer reacting from your wounds. You can be present with your partner's stress without taking it on as your own. You can parent from wisdom rather than fear. You can show up for friends without depleting yourself.

Your work becomes an expression of who you are rather than something you endure. You make decisions based on what lights you up, not what feels safest. You speak up in meetings, pursue opportunities, and trust your instincts.

Your physical health improves because your body isn't constantly flooded with stress hormones. You sleep better, digest better, and have energy for the things that matter to you.

Your creativity returns because you're not using all your mental energy to manage anxiety and overwhelm. You have space for curiosity, playfulness, and the kind of deep thinking that leads to breakthrough ideas.

Your impact on the world expands because you're no longer focused on just surviving—you're thriving. You have energy to contribute, to serve, to create something meaningful.

You were born with the capacity for all of these freedoms. They got buried under layers of stress, trauma, and survival programming. But they're still there, waiting to be uncovered.

If, as you read through the 7 Freedoms, you felt a spark of "I want that"—then you're ready.

You're ready to stop being who you've always been and discover who you actually are.

How Do You Get from Here to There? The REWIRED Process

The path from where you are to these 7 Freedoms isn't mysterious or complicated. It follows a simple pattern that I call the REWIRED Process. Every transformation in this book—every story you'll read, every shift you'll experience—follows these three steps:

1. Recognize the Reactive Loop

That moment when you catch yourself spiraling. The 3 A.M. worry fest. The pre-meeting panic. The familiar tension when that person texts. You suddenly see it: "Oh, I'm doing that thing again."

2. Interrupt with Tapping

Instead of letting the pattern run its usual course, you tap. This breaks the circuit before it can take over, and opens you up to something different.

3. Rewire Your Response

With the old pattern interrupted, your brain has space to create something new. A different reaction. A calmer default. A fresh way of responding to the same old trigger.

That's it. Recognize. Interrupt. Rewire.

This is how lasting change happens. Not through force or willpower, but through gentle, persistent repatterning of your nervous system's defaults.

Meeting You Where You Are

While Tapping has profound applications for trauma healing and deep therapeutic work, it's also something that meets you where you are, in everyday life. And this book is about Tapping for the way life actually happens.

What we're most excited about—and what we've spent years perfecting—is helping people like:

- The dad who taps in the Home Depot parking lot because hardware stores overwhelm him
- The manager who does stealth Tapping under her desk during stressful calls
- The student who taps on test anxiety between classes
- The mom who taps while hiding in the pantry for 30 seconds of peace

This isn't about replacing therapeutic work, but about giving you tools for everything that happens when you're just trying to get through the week.

The Work Is Worth It

Now, I'm not going to tell you that moving from the life you're currently living to a Rewired Life is as easy as flipping a switch. It takes showing up. It takes the courage to look at the patterns you've been avoiding. It takes the consistency to do the simple Tapping exercises in this book, even when it feels weird or you think you're "too busy."

But the work isn't another burden to add to your to-do list; it is the path to laying all those other burdens down.

The cost of staying where you are is clear—it's more of the same. More sleepless nights, more strained relationships, more days feeling like you're just surviving.

The reward for doing this work? It's not just "feeling better." It's everything. It's the life of presence, connection, and possibility that opens up when you are no longer a prisoner of your own wiring. It's the freedom to wake back up to the magical life you are meant to be living.

The question isn't whether you can change. Change is undeniably possible.

The question is: Are you willing to?

Are you willing to try?

Are you willing to consider that maybe—just maybe—the patterns that have defined your life aren't as permanent as they feel?

That's it. That's the only commitment I need from you.

Why This Matters More Than You Think

I can barely contain my excitement as I write this, because we're living in an age where neuroscience has finally caught up to what we've been seeing in practice for years. Your brain can change. Your nervous system can be rewired. Those patterns that have run your life for decades can be updated.

This isn't positive thinking. This isn't "fake it till you make it." This is biological change at the level of your nervous system.

When that woman got on the plane after 10 minutes of Tapping, she didn't overcome her fear through willpower. Her nervous system updated its response. The fear wasn't managed or coped with—it was resolved.

When the man who couldn't sleep for years due to racing thoughts finally found peace after a few weeks of Tapping, his brain didn't just learn to think positive thoughts. It rewired its stress response.

When the teacher who felt nothing after her father's death began to feel again through Tapping, she didn't force emotions. Her nervous system released from its protective freeze.

And honestly? Life is a lot more fun when you don't have to white knuckle your way through every challenge.

This should have you jumping up and down! This should have you calling your anxious friend, your sleepless partner, your fearful parent.

Because if thousands upon thousands of people have changed using this approach—why not you?

I know what's waiting for you. I've seen it thousands of times. That moment when someone realizes:

"I don't have to be anxious anymore."

"I can actually sleep."

"I can feel again."

"I'm not afraid."

"My life can change."

That moment is coming for you. Maybe in the next hour. Maybe in the next few days. But it's coming.

And when it does—when you experience your first real shift—you'll understand why I've dedicated my life to spreading this technique. You'll understand why something so simple can be so revolutionary.

Your Rewiring Journey

Here's how this is going to work:

First, I'm going to teach you the absurdly simple technique that has helped millions of people worldwide. It's going to seem too simple. You're going to wonder how tapping on your face while talking about your problems could possibly rewire your nervous system.

Then you're going to try it. Just once. It'll only take two minutes. And something is going to shift.

Maybe it'll be dramatic—like the woman who got on the plane. Maybe it'll be subtle—a slight softening of tension, a moment of unexpected calm. But something will change, and you'll think, "Huh. That's interesting."

Then I'll show you exactly why it works. The neuroscience. The research. The biological mechanisms that make this "weird tapping thing" one of the most powerful interventions available for updating your nervous system's programming.

After that, we'll dive into specific applications. Chapter by chapter, we'll address the most common human struggles. You'll learn specific protocols, hear stories of transformation, understand the science.

But more than techniques, you'll discover something profound: You have agency. You have choice. You have the power to update the patterns that have run your life.

A Note for Those Who Already Tap

Maybe you're reading this thinking, "Wait, I already know Tapping. I've been doing it for years."

Perfect. You're exactly who needs this book too.

If you've been tapping for a while, this book will take you deeper. You'll discover why some patterns seem to come back no matter how much you tap. You'll learn the neuroscience that explains what you've been experiencing. You'll get specific protocols for the stubborn stuff that hasn't shifted yet.

And you'll learn the REWIRED framework—not just releasing certain issues, but updating the entire operating system that creates them.

Plus, I'm willing to bet there are applications here you haven't tried yet. Each chapter of this book offers a window into some of the most common human struggles we *all* experience, and how to rewire those patterns using Tapping.

So consider this your next level.

How to Use This Book

Reading this book is an intervention in itself. The very act of reading it, of recognizing your patterns through the stories and reflections, begins the REWIRED process before you even do your first tap.

Your Chapter-by-Chapter Experience

Chapters 1 through 3 lay the groundwork. First you'll learn more about our family's story and how we got here, and then you'll learn all the basics of Tapping; how to do it, how it works, and the fascinating science behind it.

And then in Chapters 4 through 19, we will delve into how to apply this method in your real life.

We've identified the most common human experiences that keep people stuck—and that is what the core of this book is about.

These aren't random topics. They're the patterns we've seen over and over again after facilitating over 32 million Tapping sessions. The ones that affect nearly everyone at some point in their lives. Like when your mind won't shut up, or fear stops you cold, or other people drive you absolutely crazy.

Each of the core chapters of this book will dive into one of these experiences, helping you explore how the pattern might show up in your own life, see how others have experienced it, and understand why Tapping can help.

And then—and here's where the magic happens—you'll do a short Tapping sequence right there at the end of each chapter.

These are short Tapping experiences designed to create an immediate shift when you tap along. When you finish each chapter, you won't just understand your wiring better—you'll have already started rewiring it.

At the very back of the book, we've provided additional resources to support you, including a Tapping points guide, frequently asked questions, a deeper dive into the science and research, and more.

Why Read *Every* Chapter (Yes, Even the Ones You Don't Think Apply to You)

The patterns that run our lives show up in unexpected ways. You might not have a phobia, but the same freeze response could be why you can't speak up in meetings. You might sleep fine, but the racing mind chapter could unlock why you overthink every text message.

When we run our annual Tapping World Summit live, we cover 20 different topics, ranging from finances to relationships to insomnia. I can't count how many times someone has said, "I almost skipped that presentation because I didn't think the topic applied to me, and it ended up being my breakthrough."

Trust me on this. There's a thread through all of this that *does* apply to you—even if you don't first expect it.

The "Small Stuff" Matters

Maybe anxiety is your big challenge and motivation seems minor. Read the motivation chapter anyway. That "minor" pattern might be draining more energy than you realize—or be the key to understanding your anxiety.

This Is Also for Those You Love

Perhaps you've never experienced depression, but your partner has. Maybe phobias aren't part of your story, but they're a part of your best friend's. Each chapter helps you understand what loved ones are experiencing and gives you tools that actually help.

Future-Proof Your Nervous System

You might feel great today, but life throws curveballs.

So while you might not struggle with these specific issues today, they're all a part of the universal human experience. These chapters aren't just for current problems—they're for building resilience for whatever comes next.

I've been doing this work for 20 years, and I still discover new layers in my own patterns. I still come across new situations that reveal something new about myself and my wiring that I didn't realize before.

Think of this as your emotional first-aid kit. You wouldn't wait until you're bleeding to buy bandages. Don't wait until you're in crisis to learn these tools.

Going Deeper: The 16-Day REWIRED Challenge

Want to accelerate your transformation? At the end of each chapter, in addition to the Tapping scripts to follow along with, you'll also find a link to our 16-Day REWIRED Challenge. This allows you to take the work even deeper with guided audio sessions. Simply press Play, listen along, and immerse yourself in the Tapping experience.

Visit www.thetappingsolution.com/rewired to access all the Tapping meditations.

The Bottom Line

You picked up this book for a reason. Maybe you can name that reason clearly. Maybe it's just a feeling that something needs to change . . . that something could be different.

Either way, you're here. And that tells me you're ready to discover a fundamental truth:

You don't have to be who you've always been.

The past doesn't equal the future. Your current wiring isn't your destiny. Those patterns that feel so permanent, so "you"? They're just neural pathways that can be updated.

And they can be updated through a technique so simple a child can learn it in minutes. Through a process backed by over 300 peer-reviewed studies. Through something you can do anywhere, anytime, for free, for the rest of your life.

To be clear, this book isn't just about stopping the "bad" patterns you want to change. It's about the life that's waiting on the other side of them.

It's about reclaiming the energy you waste on anxiety so you can build the business you've been dreaming of. It's about quieting the racing thoughts so you can be truly present with your family. It's about thawing the numbness that has kept you from feeling deep love and connection. Getting REWIRED isn't just about finding peace; it's about unleashing your full power, passion, and purpose into the world.

So, are you ready to get REWIRED?

Then turn the page. Your new nervous system is waiting.

One Last Thing . . .

Before we turn the page to begin this journey, a quick note: While you'll primarily be hearing my (Nick's) voice throughout these pages, this book comes from all three of us Ortner siblings, Nick, Alex, and Jessica.

This book represents the collective work of all of us—every insight, every breakthrough, every development of this work has been a true collaboration. You'll hear Alex and Jessica's stories and perspectives woven throughout every page. We discovered this together, developed it together, and we're sharing it with you together. But for ease of reading, it'll be my voice throughout.

CHAPTER 1

Our Story

How Tapping Changed Everything

Spring 2004. I woke up with a crick in my neck so painful I could barely turn my head.

Not your normal morning stiffness—this was knife-edge, breath-catching pain.

I tried everything. Painkillers. Hot showers. Those smelly muscle rubs that make your eyes water. Nothing touched it. After days of suffering, desperate for relief, I remembered something I'd learned at a Tony Robbins event. It was this strange thing called "EFT Tapping." And I decided to try it on my neck pain.

The instructions seemed ridiculous: Tap on different points on your face and body while talking about your problem. I remember thinking, "This is either brilliantly simple or complete nonsense."

Alone in my apartment, feeling slightly silly, I started tapping my fingertips on the side of my hand, then various points on my face and chest, while saying out loud, "This pain in my neck, this terrible pain . . ."

I actually checked to make sure no one was watching through my window. The last thing I wanted was for someone to see me tapping on my face like a crazy person.

But within 10 minutes, something astonishing happened. The pain that medications hadn't touched began to dissolve. I could move my neck freely for the first time in days. I sat there, stunned into silence.

That moment changed everything.

I stood in front of my bathroom mirror, turning my head side to side, eyes wide with disbelief. The sudden absence of pain felt almost surreal—like I'd stumbled upon some hidden secret that shouldn't exist in the rational world.

It wasn't just the physical relief that floored me. It was the speed. The simplicity. The way it defied everything I thought I knew about how healing happens.

And then came the question that would reshape my entire life: "If this works for physical pain, what else could it do?"

From Personal Discovery to Global Movement

I became obsessed. And I mean *obsessed*.

The next few days, I couldn't stop thinking about what had happened. I found myself bringing it up in conversations, annoying friends and family with my newfound obsession. "Hey, I tried this weird Tapping thing, and you won't believe what happened . . ."

There was a running joke at the time, that you better not tell Nick anything's wrong, because he's going to make you tap on it.

Now, not everyone was immediately convinced like me.

I'll always remember the first time I introduced Tapping to my sister, Jessica. At the time, she was living in a small apartment with our brother, Alex, going through a career change, and dealing with a lot. And in that moment, she was sick with a cold—one of those bad colds where it just kept lingering and lingering, not getting better. I came over, and of course, thought she needed to try Tapping for it.

But as I explained how to do it, and I told her to start tapping on her face, she looked at me dubiously. "You're pranking me again, aren't you?"

You see, Jessica is the youngest of the three siblings. Growing up with two older brothers (myself and Alex), she was no stranger to having pranks played on her.

She was good natured enough to hear me out, and we did some Tapping on her cold symptoms.

But as she tapped, something shocking came out of her mouth that brought tears to her eyes: "I don't want to get better." When I asked why, she realized that being sick was the only way she could rest without drowning in guilt for not trying harder when she was already exhausted.

The symptoms were real, but there was an unconscious emotion she hadn't recognized until the Tapping quieted her mind enough to hear it. We shifted focus to tap on the crushing disappointment she felt about how life was unfolding. As soon as she honored those feelings instead of pushing through them, she felt a weight lift off her chest, and miraculously took her first deep breath in days. The congestion was completely gone.

We were both shocked.

This was just one of the countless times I was stopped in my tracks by how well this thing worked. And so I kept sharing it, with anyone and everyone I could.

What drove me wasn't just excitement about pain relief. It was a bigger realization: If I could change something as "real" as physical pain in 10 minutes, what else about myself wasn't as permanent as I believed?

That neck pain had been part of "who I was" for days. How many other parts of "who I was" were just patterns that could be updated?

And what about everyone else?

I was having this dawning realization that millions of people were suffering unnecessarily—with physical pain, anxiety, trauma, and stress—when a solution might literally be at their fingertips. People spending fortunes on treatments that barely worked. People being told their conditions were chronic and untreatable. People believing they had to live with their pain because that's just how life is.

I couldn't shake the thought: What if they're wrong? What if we all have access to a built-in healing system that most of us never learn to activate?

The Daily Life Revolution

Here's what my sister's cold story taught me: We don't need to wait for major life problems to tap. We don't need a practitioner's couch or a therapeutic breakthrough.

What we need is a tool for Tuesday at 3 P.M. when your boss sends that passive-aggressive e-mail. For Thursday night when you can't stop replaying that awkward conversation. For Sunday morning when you're dreading Monday before it even arrives.

Tapping is for **real life**—the stuff that happens between breakfast and bedtime that slowly drives us crazy.

And yes, Tapping can be brilliant for processing intense trauma or releasing deep-seated beliefs.

But what we discovered—what changed everything—is that it's also incredibly powerful as a daily tool for the thousand small moments that make up a life. Your coffee order got messed up and now you're irrationally angry? Thirty seconds of Tapping. Can't stop checking your ex's Instagram? Tap on it. Sunday scaries creeping in? Tap before they take over.

This became our specialty, our mission: making Tapping accessible for daily life. For the thousand small moments between breakfast and bedtime. For the regular Tuesday stuff that slowly drives us crazy.

We want to make Tapping so simple that you'll do it while waiting for your coffee, sitting in your car, or lying in bed unable to sleep.

The magic isn't *always* in the major breakthroughs. It's in the daily moments when you catch yourself about to spiral and choose something different.

And the best part is, it doesn't have to be complicated, or even be done perfectly, to be effective.

After Jessica first tried tapping on her cold, she forgot about it for months. That's most of us with most self-help tools, isn't it? We try something, it works, and then life gets busy . . .

Until one day, Jessica found herself back in her childhood bedroom at our parents' house after a difficult breakup, trying to cry quietly so they wouldn't hear.

She thought, "What was that Tapping thing Nick taught me?" And then she did her best to re-create it. She missed about half the points, but tapped away on herself anyway. And even just doing half of the points, she felt immediate, noticeable, physical relief. And a sense of emotional freedom—even with an imperfect technique, she was able to feel without drowning.

That's when she realized just how powerful Tapping really could be, and committed herself to learning it properly.

A Family Affair

After my sister, Jess, got on board with the whole Tapping thing, we both knew we had to share this. We knew we had to show people that we don't all have to keep going around living half lives.

But how do you tell people to tap on their faces without sounding completely insane?

Our answer: Show them.

In 2007, with maxed-out credit cards and zero filmmaking experience, we decided to make a documentary. We called it *The Tapping Solution* (originally titled *Try It on Everything*). We followed 10 people with serious issues—chronic pain, PTSD, weight struggles, phobias—and filmed what happened when they learned to tap.

The film's success surprised even us. Thousands of viewers wrote to share their own Tapping experiences.

From there, we brought the whole family into the fold. My brother, Alex, joined us as our head of marketing, our dad became our CFO, and our mom became our unpaid The Tapping Solution Foundation director. It became a true family affair to share this technique as widely as possible.

Looking back, I realize we'd been training for this our whole lives. Our mom is a therapist; our dad is an engineer.

So we had the perfect combination: one parent who understood the emotional landscape of human suffering, and another who approached problems with systematic, logical solutions.

Tapping became the bridge between these two worlds: the emotional awareness to recognize patterns and the practical tools to actually change them.

And maybe it was also the immigrant drive in our DNA that made us so determined. All three of us kids were born in Argentina before our parents brought us to the US when we were kids, and we'd grown up watching them completely rewire their lives—new country, new language, new careers, new everything.

They'd proven that transformation wasn't just possible but necessary when your current reality no longer serves you. Now we had a tool that could help people rewire their nervous systems as profoundly as our parents had rewired their entire existence.

That same willingness to leap into the unknown, to build something from nothing, to transform completely—it's what drove us to max out those credit cards and make that documentary.

So, what started as a grassroots movement grew into our first Tapping World Summit in 2009, which reached over 50,000 people online. Today, that annual event reaches over 500,000 participants worldwide year after year.

Alex, Jess, and I now run The Tapping Solution App. We've written bestselling books, we've presented on major stages and TV shows like *TODAY*, Dr. Oz, the *Tamron Hall Show*, and more. We've reached millions of people with our message.

But honestly? We're still just three siblings who discovered something that worked and couldn't stop sharing it.

In fact, we often joke that Tapping *must* work, because no one can get on your nerves like your own family, and yet we managed to create a thriving family business together.

The Moment We Knew This Was Bigger Than Us

December 14, 2012. Sandy Hook Elementary School. Newtown, Connecticut.

Our hometown.

Twenty children and six educators killed. Our small, quiet community shattered. The world watched in horror, but we lived it. These were our neighbors, our friends, our community.

In those first dark days, Jessica, Alex, and I huddled together, asking the same question everyone was asking: "What can we do?"

We had this tool. This strange, simple technique that helped with trauma. But how could Tapping possibly help with something this devastating?

I'll never forget sitting with Scarlett Lewis just days after her six-year-old son, Jesse, was killed in the shooting. The weight of her grief was unbearable to witness. But she was open to trying anything that might help her breathe through the next moment.

As we tapped together through unimaginable pain, she felt what she later described as "the first lifting of the weight on my chest." Not erasing her loss—nothing could do that—but creating just enough space to take a breath.

"It was the first moment since Jesse died that I felt I might survive this," she told me later.

That's when we knew. This wasn't just about fixing everyday stress or helping people sleep better. This was about giving people a tool to survive the worst moments of their lives and eventually find their way back to hope.

In our darkest moment as a community, Tapping gave us something precious: agency. We couldn't change what happened. But we could reclaim our power to choose how we responded to it.

We established The Tapping Solution Foundation to bring trauma relief to our community. We trained counselors, teachers, parents. We worked with first responders who carried images they couldn't unsee.

Scarlett went on to found the Choose Love Movement, reaching millions with social-emotional learning. She credits Tapping as one of the tools that helped her transform her grief into purpose.

That tragedy taught us something profound: When you discover something that truly helps, you have a responsibility to share it. Not because it's a business. Not because it's interesting. But because somewhere, someone is suffering, and they deserve to know that relief is possible.

The Ripple Effect

Every day, we get e-mails. Thousands of them. Each one reminds us why we do this work.

The veteran who wrote: "Last night I slept all the way through for the first time in 20-plus years. When I started using this Tapping meditation, I was waking five times a night, so it's caused a massive improvement."

The mother who shared: "Creating new and lasting habits is something that I've traditionally struggled with. With Tapping I am generally calmer and find it easier to manage upsetting incidences and to reset after an upset. My relationships with my significant other and my kids are much calmer and more meaningful."

The 50-year-old woman who confessed: "I have to say this really created a positive shift in my mindset and helped release trauma, anger, and anxiety that was keeping me from living life. I feel alive. I see things differently, like a curtain has been pulled away from my mind's eye. Oh the possibilities of living!"

Each person had accepted their struggle as common for someone in their situation, as "just how it is." And each discovered it didn't have to be.

Every. Single. Story. Matters.

And here's what really keeps us going: the ripple effect.

That mother who stopped screaming? Her kids are learning to tap when they're upset. The veteran who found peace? He's teaching other vets. The executive who overcame anxiety? She introduced Tapping to her entire company.

Each person who discovers Tapping becomes a messenger. Not because we ask them to, but because when you find something that changes your life, you can't help but share it.

What This Means for You

I know what you might be thinking, because I thought it too: "Sure, it worked for them, but my situation is different."

I get it. I really do.

When I first learned about Tapping, I thought: "This might work for other people, but I'm too logical/skeptical/messed up/unique for something this simple."

But here's what 20 years of this work has taught me: Everyone thinks they're the exception. The CEO thinks her stress is more complex than everyone else's. The trauma survivor thinks his pain is too deep. The anxious mom thinks her worry is never going anywhere.

And then they tap. And something shifts.

Not because they're special or because they did it perfectly. But because this technique works at a level deeper than our stories about why we're stuck.

Your nervous system doesn't care if you're a skeptic or a believer. It doesn't care if you're a CEO or a student, a veteran or a teacher. When you tap, you're speaking directly to the part of your brain that controls your stress response. And that part responds.

You don't need to believe me. You don't need to trust the science (though there's plenty, and I'll certainly share some of it with you). You don't even need to hope it will work.

You just need to try it.

Your Story Starts Now

Twenty years ago, I was just a guy with neck pain who stumbled onto something weird on the Internet.

Today, along with my siblings Alex and Jessica, we've helped facilitate over 32 million Tapping sessions worldwide through one-on-one coaching, group sessions, and via our app.

All these years later, I sometimes think about alternate-universe Nick—the one who stayed stuck with that neck pain, who never discovered Tapping, who kept living the same patterns.

He'd probably still be stressed, still be searching, still believing that some struggles are just part of life. He'd never know about the freedoms waiting for him on the other side of his current wiring.

But that's not my story. And it doesn't have to be yours.

Right now, you're where I was that morning with the neck pain. You have a choice: Keep doing what you've always done—pushing through, accepting that "this is just how it is," doing the same old things day after day. Or try something different.

Something that seems too simple. Something that might just change everything. I know which choice changed my life.

Your story, your breakthrough, is waiting on the next page. The technique that changed our lives, that helped our community heal from unimaginable tragedy, that has transformed millions of lives around the world, is about to become yours.

Once you experience that first shift—that moment when your stress drops, your racing thoughts quiet, your body relaxes—you'll understand why we can't stop sharing this.

You'll understand why something so simple can be so revolutionary.

And maybe, just maybe, you'll become one of those people who can't help but share it too. Not because you have to, but because when you discover something that truly helps, keeping it to yourself feels impossible.

Ready to experience what changed our lives?

Let's learn how to tap.

CHAPTER 2

Your First Tap

A Simple Practice with Profound Power

The technique you're about to learn involves tapping on your face with your fingertips while focusing on what's bothering you. Yes, it looks weird. Yes, you might feel silly at first.

But if you actually try it instead of just reading about it, something is going to shift.

Something will change. And you'll think, "Wait . . . what just happened?"

What happened is you just hacked into your nervous system and told it to chill out. In about two minutes. With your fingertips.

So let's dive in!

Before We Start: Where Are You Right Now?

Before I show you how to tap, let's capture where you are in this exact moment. This isn't a test; it's just helpful to know where you're starting so you can notice what changes.

Take a breath and scan through these questions:

- What's your mind doing right now? Racing? Foggy? Skeptical? Curious?

- What's your body feeling? Tense? Tired? Numb? Agitated?
- How long have you been feeling this way? Hours? Days? Years?
- If you had to rate your overall stress level from 0 to 10 (with 10 being maximum stress), what number comes to mind?
- Is there a specific thing bothering you right now? A worry, a physical discomfort, an emotion?

Just notice. Don't try to fix or change anything. We're just taking a snapshot of this moment.

Got it? Good. Now let's learn this technique that's helped millions of people, from combat veterans to Olympic athletes, from anxious kids to Fortune 500 CEOs.

The Basic Recipe: How to Tap

Tapping (also known as EFT—Emotional Freedom Techniques, a name that captures both the technique and its goal: emotional freedom) combines two simple elements that create profound change:

1. **Physical tapping** on specific acupressure points on your body
2. **Focused attention** on what's bothering you

That's it. No special equipment. No apps required (though we have one if you want guided sessions). No previous experience necessary.

Here's what makes this powerful (and we'll go into this way deeper in the next chapter): When you think about something stressful, your body normally tenses up and your brain sounds the alarm. But when you tap on these specific points while thinking about that stressor, you're sending calming signals to your brain at the same time.

Your brain gets confused—in the best way. It's registering the problem but receiving safety signals. In that contradiction, it can finally update its response.

The 9 Tapping Points

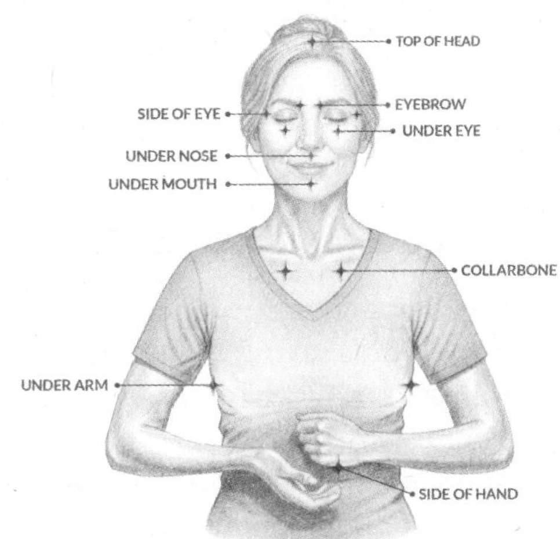

1. **Side of the Hand**—Between the base of the pinky finger and the wrist, along the fleshy, narrow side of the hand
2. **Eyebrow**—Where your eyebrow begins, near the bridge of your nose
3. **Side of the Eye**—On the bone at the outer side of your eye
4. **Under the Eye**—On the bone directly under your eye
5. **Under the Nose**—Between your nose and upper lip
6. **Under the Mouth**—In the crease between your lower lip and chin
7. **Collarbone**—Feel for the two little bones of the collarbone and go down and out about an inch on each side
8. **Under the Arm**—About four inches (or a hand's width) below your armpit
9. **Top of the Head**—Right on the crown of the head

If you need a quick reminder of the Tapping points at any time, you can find an easy guide and diagram by flipping to page 295 in Appendix A.

Here's the basic recipe:

Step 1: Pick Your Target

What's bugging you right now? Be specific. Instead of "I'm stressed," try:

- "This tension in my shoulders"
- "I can't stop thinking about that meeting"
- "This anxiety about my kids"
- "I'm exhausted but can't relax"

Step 2: Rate the Intensity

On a scale of 0 to 10, how intense is this issue right now? Don't overthink it, just go with your first instinct.

Step 3: The Setup Statement

We start by tapping on the **side of the hand point**, the fleshy part on the side of your hand, while saying a setup statement three times. The setup statement is designed to acknowledge the issue and help neutralize any judgments you have around your experience.

A setup statement might sound like:

"Even though [your specific issue], I acknowledge how I feel."

For example:

- "Even though I have this tension in my shoulders, I acknowledge how I feel."
- "Even though I can't stop worrying about tomorrow's presentation, I choose to be kind to myself anyway."
- "Even though I feel completely overwhelmed right now, I accept how I'm feeling in this moment."

Say it three times while continuously tapping the side of your hand.

Step 4: The Tapping Sequence

Now we tap through the rest of the points while focusing on the issue. You can tap with either hand, on either side of your body or on both sides at the same time (the acupressure points are symmetrical). Use 1 to 3 fingertips and tap firmly but gently, like you're drumming on a table.

As you tap through the points, we often use phrases to help us stay focused on the emotion or experience we are trying to let go of. You can do that by either giving words to how you're feeling like you are sharing it with a friend, or you can repeat one simple phrase to help you stay focused. This could sound like:

- "This shoulder tension"
- "This worry"
- "All this stress"
- "Can't relax"

Keep tapping through the points until you feel a shift and more ease. When you find yourself being able to think a positive thought without being resistant to it, you can shift to saying more empowering statements.

This is where the rewiring happens. You focus on releasing the old pattern (like weeding in a garden), to make room to plant something more empowering.

Step 5: Check In Again

Once you feel a great sense of release, stop tapping and take a deep breath. Check in with yourself. What's your number now? Has anything shifted?

That's the basic recipe. Simple, right? Want more guidance, and need to see the process in action? You can find more information and a video tap-along guide at www.thetappingsolution.com/rewired.

Why These Specific Points? A Quick Word About Meridians

You'll often hear the Tapping points referred to as "acupressure points" or "meridian points." And it's true, they are some of the same points used in acupressure (or acupuncture, minus the needles). That language comes from traditional Chinese medicine, which described the body as having channels—or meridians—through which life force energy flows.

Meridians are believed to be connected to various organs and bodily functions. When the acupressure points along these channels are stimulated—whether through acupuncture needles, finger pressure, or Tapping—it can help balance the body's energy flow, alleviate physical discomfort or emotional distress, and promote healing.

Modern research now suggests that these points align closely with nerve bundles and connective tissue pathways that directly communicate with the brain and the body's stress circuits. So while ancient healers described this in terms of "energy," we can now understand it as part of your body's intricate communication network.

In other words, when you tap, you're not doing something mystical—you're engaging your nervous system in a very real, measurable way.

Common Questions Before We Give It a Try

"Do I have to say those exact words?" No. The words are just to keep you focused on the issue. Use whatever words feel true for you.

"Why am I focusing on the negative?" When you tap while acknowledging what's actually happening for you (the stress, the fear, the frustration, the symptom), you're telling your brain: "I see you, I hear you, and it's safe to release this now." As we acknowledge the truth of what we're feeling while calming our nervous system with Tapping, we help to neutralize the old pattern so we can finally let it go.

"When do I move to the positive?" Once you've released some of the "charge" of the issue, you can begin to move toward more empowering statements that open up to new, more positive possibilities. When you can think about the issue without that tight chest, racing thoughts, or sick feeling in your stomach, that's when your nervous system is ready to install something new. It's like weeding a garden; only when you've cleared enough away can you begin to plant new seeds. This is where the rewiring process really happens—we release the old pattern and begin to install the new wiring.

"Can I ever just focus on the positive?" Absolutely! If you're already feeling calm and at ease, it's a great time to focus your Tapping entirely on the positive. From a calm centered place, Tapping helps positive beliefs, thoughts, and feelings take deep root.

"What's the difference between me tapping on my own and a guided Tapping meditation?" Think of it like this: Some people like to cook using a recipe, and some like to wing it based on what feels right in the moment. Sometimes it's nice to just follow instructions, and sometimes it's nice to just do your own thing.

"Do I tap hard or soft?" Firm but gentle. Like you're drumming your fingers when impatient, or like a woodpecker on a tree.

"Which side do I tap on?" Either side works. The acupressure points used in Tapping exist on both sides of your body. If you can tap on both sides at the same time, do it! If not, you can choose one side or switch between them. It's up to you.

"Can I do this wrong?" The only way to do it wrong is to not do it at all. We want to hit the actual points as accurately as possible (try not to tap in the middle of your forehead, that's not one of the points!), but don't stress about it. Even imperfect Tapping works better than perfect worrying.

"What if I feel silly doing this?" Join the club. Everyone feels silly at first. I hid from my roommates. My sister thought I was pranking her. CEOs do this in bathroom stalls. Parents hide in closets to tap. You know what's sillier? Staying stressed because you're too embarrassed to tap your face for a few minutes. There's always a way—if you need to tap in the bathroom, or sitting in your car? Do it.

Finding *Your* Path to Self-Acceptance

The phrase "I deeply and completely love and accept myself" is used in the **traditional setup statement** in EFT Tapping. Its purpose is powerful: to introduce the idea of self-acceptance right when you're focused on a problem. The goal is to quiet the internal critic and calm the nervous system's fight against itself, which is a crucial part of the healing process. What we resist, persists, but what we accept can move through us.

However, we recognize that when you're overwhelmed by anxiety, pain, or self-judgment, that phrase can feel like a big leap. And forcing yourself to say something that feels inauthentic can create more resistance, which is the opposite of what we want.

Think of self-acceptance as the destination. While the traditional phrase is a direct route, there are many other avenues to get there. The following are some options we've found for statements that can help you move in that direction without as much internal resistance:

- "I acknowledge how I feel."
- "I accept how I'm feeling in this moment."
- "I choose to be kind to myself anyway."
- "I give my body permission to relax."

All these paths lead to the same destination. The words are not a magic spell; they are a tool to bring kindness and acceptance to your struggle. Choose the path that feels most available and true for you today.

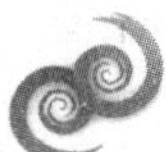

TAPPING SCRIPT: *Your First Two-Minute Stress Relief Tap*

Okay, enough reading about it. Let's actually do this.

First, think about whatever is causing you the most stress right now. Got it? Rate it from 0 to 10.

Now, tap on the side of your hand and repeat this statement three times.

Side of the Hand: Even though I'm feeling all this stress and tension, I acknowledge how I feel.

Then tap through each point while saying these phrases out loud or in your mind:

Eyebrow: This feeling of stress
Side of the Eye: Feeling overwhelmed
Under the Eye: Too much going on
Under the Nose: All this pressure
Under the Mouth: This stress in my body
Collarbone: My racing mind
Under the Arm: It's okay to begin to slow down . . .
Top of the Head: and notice how I feel

Eyebrow: Maybe I can relax a little more right now
Side of the Eye: I'm safe in this moment
Under the Eye: It's okay to take a break
Under the Nose: It's okay to release this tension
Under the Mouth: I am interrupting this stress loop . . .
Collarbone: and choosing something new
Under the Arm: Opening up to greater ease
Top of the Head: Sending calming signals to my nervous system

Eyebrow: It's safe to let go
Side of the Eye: Allowing my body to soften
Under the Eye: Allowing my mind to settle
Under the Nose: Breathing more deeply
Under the Mouth: Feeling grounded and present

Collarbone: As I give myself this moment to reset,
Under the Arm: I open up to a new sense of possibility
Top of the Head: I am calm, centered, and ready for what's next

Now stop. Breathe. Check in with yourself.

What's your stress number now? What feels different in your body? What's shifted in your mind?

"Did That Actually Just Work?"

If you just did the Tapping instead of just reading about it, you probably noticed something change. Maybe:

- Your shoulders dropped
- Your breathing deepened
- Your mind felt clearer
- The intensity of your stress decreased
- You felt a wave of calm (or maybe emotion)
- You yawned or sighed (signs of nervous system relaxation)

Or maybe you felt silly tapping on your face and are wondering if you're just imagining the shift.

Here's what I want you to know: You're not imagining it. Something real just happened in your nervous system. In the next chapter I'll explain exactly what and why. But for now, just notice that in two minutes, using nothing but your fingertips and your attention, you changed your state.

Let me be direct about what just happened: You just proved you have more control over your internal state than you've been taught to believe.

That's the power you're holding in your hands—literally.

You have agency. You have choice. You have the power to shift your state whenever you need to.

How does it feel to discover you've been carrying the solution with you all along?

The Invitation

You now know how to tap. It took you maybe 10 minutes to learn and 2 minutes to experience. You have a tool that:

- Requires no equipment
- Costs nothing
- Can be done anywhere
- Works in minutes
- Has zero side effects
- Gets more effective with practice

But here's the thing: Knowing how to tap and actually Tapping are two different things. It's like knowing that exercise is good for you versus actually moving your body.

So here's my invitation: For the next 24 hours, whenever you feel stress, anxiety, frustration, or any uncomfortable emotion, take a few minutes and tap. Use the simple script I just gave you, or make up your own words.

Just tap. See what happens.

Because while I can tell you stories of transformation, cite research studies, and explain mechanisms all day long (and I will in Part B), nothing will convince you like your own experience.

You've spent years, maybe decades, being wired a certain way. In the last few minutes, you just started the rewiring process.

How does it feel to know you have that power?

What Becomes Possible Now

So, you've learned the technique. You've (hopefully) tried it. Maybe you've even felt something (even a small thing) shift.

But let me paint you a picture of what this really means:

Tonight, when your mind starts racing, you have options.

Tomorrow, when stress hijacks your morning, you can interrupt it.

Next week, when that situation triggers you again, you can rewire your response.

Next month, you might notice you're not getting triggered at all.

This isn't about becoming someone new. It's about no longer being controlled by old wiring you didn't choose.

You just took your first step from "this is just how I am" to "I can change this."

Keep Tapping. Keep rewiring. Your new nervous system is already under construction.

What's Next?

Now you might be wondering: How can something so simple create real change? What's actually happening in my brain and body when I tap? Why does acknowledging negative feelings while tapping somehow make them dissolve?

Those are exactly the right questions. And in the next chapter, I'm going to answer them with science, stories, and a deeper understanding of why this "weird tapping thing" might just be the most powerful tool you'll ever learn for rewiring your nervous system.

But first, go tap on something else. Right now. Pick any minor annoyance in your life and spend a couple of minutes tapping on it.

Because the more you experience this working, the more your skeptical mind will quiet down and let the transformation really begin.

Ready to understand why this works? Turn the page.

CHAPTER 3

The Science of Rewiring

What's Really Happening in Your Brain and Body

So you just tapped on your face for two minutes and something shifted. Your stress went from a 7 to a 4. That chatter of worry in your mind quieted down. The tension in your shoulders released.

And now your logical mind is doing gymnastics trying to figure out what just happened.

"Was it just distraction?" "Is this some kind of placebo effect?" "Did I just imagine feeling better?" "How could something so simple actually work?"

Maybe you're the person who reads every study before trying something new. Or the one who's been burned by promises of "instant transformation." Or you're just tired of hoping. I see you.

I get it. It's natural to feel skeptical. I had the same thoughts when I first discovered Tapping. It seemed too simple, too weird, too good to be true.

That's the exact same reaction a psychologist named Dr. Callahan had when he first discovered the technique.

The Accidental Discovery That Defied Everything We Knew About Healing

The story begins in 1980 with psychologist Dr. Roger Callahan and his patient Mary.

Mary had such severe water phobia that she couldn't take baths, couldn't go near swimming pools, and had nightmares about drowning. For 18 months, Dr. Callahan tried every technique in his arsenal: systematic desensitization, cognitive therapy, hypnosis. Nothing worked.

One afternoon, Mary mentioned that whenever she thought about water, she felt a terrible sensation in her stomach. Dr. Callahan had recently been studying traditional Chinese medicine and knew there was an acupuncture point under the eye connected to the stomach meridian.

On an impulse, he asked Mary to tap under her eye while thinking about water.

What happened next made no sense: Her expression changed dramatically, and she looked at Dr. Callahan. "It's gone!" she said. "That awful feeling in the pit of my stomach—it's completely gone!"

They were both perplexed by a result neither was expecting.

Mary immediately went outside to Dr. Callahan's swimming pool to test her fear, and as she sat on the edge, she felt . . . completely okay. That night, she took the test even further and went to the beach. And the change had stuck.

Mary's lifelong phobia had vanished. Instantly.

Mary had been "someone with a water phobia" for her entire life. It was part of her identity, her story, who she was. Her family knew it. Her friends accommodated it. She built her life around it.

In 30 seconds, she discovered a profound truth: She didn't have to be "someone with a water phobia" anymore.

That identity, "person with water phobia," wasn't who she was. It was just how she was wired. And wiring can be changed.

"This Can't Be Real"

Dr. Callahan's colleagues thought he'd lost his mind. A patient doesn't overcome a severe phobia by tapping on her face for just a few minutes. It violated everything they knew about how psychology worked.

But Mary didn't care about psychological theory. She was free.

And she wasn't alone. As Dr. Callahan refined his approach (which at the time he called Thought Field Therapy), the "impossible" results kept happening. Phobias dissolving in minutes. Trauma symptoms disappearing. Anxiety vanishing.

His student, Gary Craig, simplified the technique into EFT (Emotional Freedom Techniques), making it accessible to everyone. And that's when things got really interesting.

Millions of people started Tapping. Combat veterans overcame PTSD. Accident victims released trauma. People with lifelong anxiety found peace. The anecdotal evidence was overwhelming, and it started sneaking into academia, but science remained skeptical.

How could tapping on your face change your brain? It took decades of research to answer that question. And the answer revolutionizes our understanding of how change happens.

But first, to really understand the power of what's happening, we need to look at your body's electrical system.

Your Body's Electrical System

Think of your body like a house with electrical wiring. When everything's working right, the lights turn on, the appliances run, everything flows.

But what happens when there's a short circuit? The lights flicker. Breakers trip. Things stop working properly.

That's what trauma and chronic stress do to your body's electrical system. They create short circuits that keep triggering the same responses over and over:

- See a dog → panic (even though one dog bit you 20 years ago)
- Read e-mail from boss → stomach knots (even though you're good at your job)
- Think about money → chest tightens (even though you're not actually in danger)

Can you see yourself in any of these or something similar? These are your short circuits in action.

Traditional therapy helps you understand these patterns, like having an electrician explain why your circuits keep tripping. This understanding is incredibly valuable. It gives you insight, context, and often profound awareness about why you react the way you do.

But Tapping does something different, and can often accelerate results to the next level. It resets your body's electrical system by stimulating specific points that send calming signals directly to your brain's alarm center.

The Memory Update Phenomenon

Here's where it gets really cool. Scientists discovered something amazing: When you remember something, that memory becomes temporarily "unlocked" and changeable, like opening a document on your computer.

For a short window of time after recalling a memory, you can actually edit it before it gets saved again.

This is why Mary's water phobia could vanish in minutes. When she thought about water (opened the file) while tapping (added new information), her brain actually updated the memory. The next time she thought about water, the fear was gone because the memory itself had been changed.

Think about that. You're not learning to cope with fear. You're actually updating the source code.

The Reactive Loops Running Your Life

Every day, your brain runs thousands of automatic programs. Think of them like your phone's apps running in the background—except these apps control your reactions, emotions, and behaviors.

These aren't flaws. They're actually your brain trying to protect you based on past experiences.

Here's how it works: Something bad happens once, and your brain goes, "Got it. I'll make sure we're ready if that happens again." It creates an automatic response—a shortcut to keep you safe.

The problem? Your brain is terrible at updating these programs. That presentation that went badly in high school? Your brain still thinks every presentation is a threat. That relationship that ended painfully? Your brain tenses up around every new connection.

I call these outdated programs "Reactive Loops," automatic stress responses that fire without your permission. Each loop has three parts: a trigger (what sets it off), an automatic response (what happens in your body and mind), and a predictable result (how it hijacks your life).

Examples of common Reactive Loops include:

- Racing thoughts at 3 A.M. when you can't sleep (your brain thinks worrying keeps you safe)
- Anxiety before social events (your brain remembers that one awkward party)

- Procrastination on important tasks (your brain recalls when trying led to criticism)
- Tension around certain people (your brain hasn't forgotten old hurts)

These loops feel permanent because they've carved pathways in your brain through repetition. It's like water flowing down a hillside; it naturally follows the deepest groove.

This is part of what I call the Great Forgetting—a collective amnesia about what's actually possible for human beings. We've forgotten that these grooves aren't permanent. We've accepted our racing minds, our hair-trigger reactions, our chronic exhaustion as "just who we are."

We've forgotten what it feels like to have a quiet mind, a calm body, authentic energy. We've forgotten these are our birthright, not special occasions.

Just because everyone you know has these patterns doesn't mean they're mandatory human experiences.

These patterns can be changed. Scientists call it neuroplasticity; I call it hope.

The Familiarity Trap

Here's the weird part: We stay stuck in painful patterns because they're familiar. And to your brain, familiar equals safe, even when it's making you miserable.

It's like staying in a bad relationship because at least you know what to expect. Or keeping a job you hate because the devil you know feels safer than the unknown.

Your brain would rather repeat a familiar pattern that makes you anxious than risk trying something new. That's the Familiarity Trap—your brain's tendency to choose the known (even if it's miserable) over unknown possibility.

This explains why:

- Knowing better doesn't automatically lead to doing better
- You can read all the self-help books and still repeat the same patterns
- Logic alone can't override these deep grooves in your brain

And the cost? Let's be honest:

- Relationships that never deepen because you're always braced for hurt
- Opportunities missed because "that's not who I am"

- Dreams deferred because the familiar feels safer than the possible
- A life lived at 60 percent because 100 percent feels too risky

You're paying this price every single day. Not because you have to, but because your brain thinks familiar suffering is safer than unfamiliar freedom.

So how do you escape the trap?

PAUSE *and* REFLECT

Take a moment. What's one painful-but-familiar pattern you keep finding yourself falling into? What's one pattern that feels familiar but is coming at a cost? Maybe it's related to a job, a relationship dynamic, a way of thinking about yourself?

The Choice Point

Every time you face a trigger, you hit what I call a "Choice Point." In that split second, you either:

1. **Fall into your Reactive Loop** (the old automatic response)
2. **Choose something new**

Without a tool to help you, you'll almost always choose door #1. It's the path of least resistance, the superhighway in your brain versus the overgrown dirt path of something new.

But Tapping changes the game. It gives you a way to choose door #2, even when every cell in your body wants to run the old program. And when you choose door #2, you create what I call a Rewired Response: a new, calmer pattern that replaces your old Reactive Loop.

A Rewired Response feels different in your body. Where you used to tense up, you stay soft. Where your mind used to race, it stays curious. Same situation, completely different internal experience.

And here's the beautiful part: Each time you choose this new response, it gets easier. You're building new neural highways that will eventually become as automatic as your old patterns, except these ones lead somewhere you actually want to go.

A Review of the REWIRED Process: The 3 Steps That Change Everything

Now that you understand both the how and the why, let me return to the framework that ties this whole book together.

Remember that simple three-step process I introduced at the beginning of this book? Recognize. Interrupt. Rewire.

John with his insomnia, Erin with her anxiety and depression, Mary with her water phobia . . . they all followed the same three steps, whether they realized it or not.

And now you—you have the fundamentals to understand *why* it works:

1. When you **Recognize** a Reactive Loop, you're catching your brain running its automatic stress program
2. When you **Interrupt** with Tapping, you're breaking the stress circuit and confusing your nervous system (in a good way!)
3. When you **Rewire**, you're taking advantage of that confusion to teach your brain a new, calmer response

This is how lasting change happens. Not through force or willpower, but through gentle, persistent rewiring of your nervous system's defaults.

This isn't just a framework; it's your new superpower. The ability to catch yourself mid-spiral and choose a different response. The power to update patterns that have run your life for years.

Throughout this book, you'll see these three steps in action. With real people and their real stories. No matter the context, no matter the individual, each story follows a similar pattern.

In each chapter that follows, you'll learn to recognize specific Reactive Loops:

- The mental spin cycles (Chapter 5)
- The motivation flatline (Chapter 10)
- The inner critic assault (Chapter 11)
- And many more

For each one, I'll show you exactly how to interrupt it with Tapping and what your Rewired Response can look like.

But remember: This isn't about perfection. You won't catch every loop. You won't interrupt every pattern. And that's completely fine.

Even catching and rewiring 10 percent of your Reactive Loops will transform your life. Because each time you do it, you prove to your nervous system that change is possible.

The Agency I Never Knew I Had

For most of my early life, I moved through the world like a passenger on a train I hadn't chosen to board. Things just . . . happened. Good days happened. Bad days happened. I got angry, I got happy, I got stressed . . . all of it just washing over me like weather I couldn't control.

I genuinely believed this was how life worked. You wake up, life happens *to* you, you react however you react, you go to bed. Repeat.

Looking back now, I can see I was trapped in endless Reactive Loops, those automatic stress responses firing all day long.

Then I discovered Tapping, and with it came a revelation that fundamentally rewired how I understood my own life: I wasn't just a passenger. I had a say in how I responded to what happened around me.

The shift was quiet but profound. And it was gradual. No one else could see it, but inside, I was slowly changing.

I began to understand that while I couldn't control all the events of my life, I could control how I participated in them. I could respond with intention rather than just ricochet off circumstances like a pinball. I began catching myself at what I now call Choice Points: those split seconds where I could either fall into my usual reaction or try something different.

This wasn't about positive thinking or forcing myself to feel differently. It was about discovering I actually had agency in my own emotional life. That I could choose to tap instead of spiral. That I could interrupt old patterns instead of being at their mercy.

What I didn't realize at the time was that I was creating Rewired Responses. I was creating new, calmer patterns to replace the Reactive Loops that had run my life.

This was the end to my personal Great Forgetting. I remembered that these patterns weren't my identity; they were just my wiring. And wiring can be changed.

Discovering I could rewire these "natural" responses? That changed everything.

How Tapping Rewires Your Brain: The 5 Core Principles

Three hundred studies and 32 million completed Tapping sessions in our app later, we've discovered exactly why this works. Here are the five principles that create such profound change:

1. Breaking the Brain's Reactive Loops

Your brain plays the same stress patterns on repeat, like a broken record. Tapping physically interrupts these loops, giving your brain a chance to play a different song. Without this interruption, the same patterns run your life on autopilot.

2. Safety + Awareness = Transformation

Here's the magic combination: You focus on what bothers you (awareness), while Tapping sends calming signals to your body (safety). Your brain gets confused: "Wait, I'm thinking about this scary thing, but I feel calm?" This confusion forces it to update old programming.

3. Processing Through the Body, Not Just the Mind

You can't think your way out of feelings—they live in your body. Tapping gives emotions a physical pathway to finally complete and release. That's why people often cry, yawn, or feel tingling while tapping. It's emotions finally moving out instead of staying stuck.

4. Resetting Your Nervous System

Your body has two modes: "Go" (stress) and "Rest" (healing). Most of us are stuck in "Go" mode 24/7. Tapping flips the switch to "Rest" mode, where actual change happens. It tells your nervous system: "You can chill now."

5. Repetition Rewires the Brain

Your current patterns got strong through repetition. Tapping uses this same principle in reverse. Each time you tap instead of spiral, you build new neural pathways of calm. Eventually, calm becomes your new default instead of stress.

These five principles don't just explain how Tapping works; they're your pathway to the 7 Freedoms of a Rewired Life. Remember these from the Introduction?

1. **The ability to experience emotional freedom**—emotions flow through you instead of taking you down. You can feel without drowning and think without spiraling

2. **The ability to respond rather than react**—space between trigger and response, choice where there was only reflex
3. **The ability to feel calm in situations that used to throw you**—not fake Zen, actual nervous system regulation
4. **The ability to access energy you didn't know you had**—your cellular power plants working properly again
5. **The ability to feel at home in your body**—physical ease as normal, not exceptional
6. **The ability to trust yourself to handle whatever comes**—uncertainty becomes interesting, not terrifying
7. **The ability to show up as your *real* self**—instead of who you've always been or who you think you *should* be

When you break Reactive Loops driven by stress, you gain emotional freedom.

When you create safety while processing, you develop the ability to respond rather than react.

When you reset your nervous system, you feel at home in your body.

When you rewire through repetition, you trust yourself to handle whatever comes.

Each Tapping session builds your capacity for the life waiting on the other side of your current wiring.

Your Brain's Command Center: A Quick Introduction

Before we go further, let me introduce you to the key players in your stress response—the parts of your brain and body that Tapping directly influences. Don't worry, this isn't going to be a biology lecture. Just think of it as meeting the cast of characters in your nervous system's daily drama.

The Autonomic Nervous System: Your Two-Mode Operating System

Let's start with the big picture. Your body runs on two primary settings, controlled by a branch of your nervous system called the *autonomic nervous system*:

- **Sympathetic Mode ("Go"/"Fight-or-Flight"):** This is your body's gas pedal. Heart rate speeds up, breathing gets shallow, muscles tense, digestion shuts down. Great mode for responding to actual emergencies. Terrible when it's running 24/7 because your brain thinks every little thing is a threat. This is where those Reactive Loops live—in constant sympathetic activation.
- **Parasympathetic Mode ("Rest"/"Rest-and-Digest"):** This is your body's brake pedal. Heart rate slows, breathing deepens, muscles relax, healing systems activate. This is the mode where you can think clearly instead of just reacting. Where you have space to make different choices at those Choice Points we talked about. Where your nervous system can actually create Rewired Responses instead of just running the same old loops.

And in some situations, we can also drop into a shutdown or "freeze" response (like a deep "brake" that's different from relaxed rest).

The Limbic System and Amygdala: What Controls the Gas Pedal

Now let's zoom in. What's actually in charge of triggering that fight-or-flight response mentioned in the last section?

Deep in your brain sits a collection of structures called the limbic system—your emotional processing center. This is where feelings get created, memories get emotionally tagged, and your survival instincts live.

Within the limbic system lives the amygdala, a small almond-shaped structure (about the size of, well, an almond) that serves as your brain's threat detection system. Your amygdala has one job: scan everything for danger and sound the alarm when it finds a threat. Think of it as your internal smoke detector, but one with a hair-trigger sensitivity and a really long memory.

The HPA Axis: The Stress Highway System

When your amygdala hits that alarm, it activates what scientists call the **HPA axis** (Hypothalamic-Pituitary-Adrenal axis). Think of it as a highway system carrying stress signals throughout your entire body.

Here's the route: Your hypothalamus (the command center) sends an urgent message to your pituitary gland (the messenger), which tells your adrenal glands to flood your bloodstream with stress hormones—which help your body prepare to fight or flee.

The main stress hormone? *Cortisol*—the chemical that makes you feel simultaneously wired and exhausted. It's what's coursing through your system when you're anxious, when you can't sleep at 3 A.M., when you're overwhelmed by your to-do list.

The Prefrontal Cortex: Your Wise Advisor

Behind your forehead sits your prefrontal cortex–your rational, planning brain. When stress activates your amygdala, blood flow decreases to this thinking brain. That's why you can't think clearly when you're panicking, why you say things you regret when you're angry, why you make questionable decisions when you're stressed–your wise advisor is offline.

Tapping restores communication between your emotional brain and thinking brain, so you can respond thoughtfully instead of reacting automatically.

The Chemical Messengers: Your Neurotransmitters

Finally, let's talk about your **neurotransmitters**–the chemical messengers that profoundly influence how you feel:

- **Serotonin:** Your mood stabilizer and contentment chemical (low levels linked to depression)
- **Dopamine:** Your motivation and reward chemical (the "I want to do things" feeling)
- **Norepinephrine:** Your alertness and focus chemical (great in small doses, anxiety-producing in excess)
- **GABA:** Your calming chemical that puts the brakes on anxiety and racing thoughts

When these chemicals are balanced, you feel good–motivated but not manic, alert but not anxious, content but not numb. When they're out of whack–often due to chronic stress repeatedly activating that HPA axis–you end up anxious, sad, unmotivated, or exhausted. Or all of the above.

How It All Connects

Here's the beautiful part: When you stimulate specific acupressure points while Tapping, you're not just addressing one piece of this system. You're influencing the entire network.

You're calming your amygdala, interrupting the HPA axis, shifting from sympathetic to parasympathetic mode, reconnecting your prefrontal cortex, and helping restore balance to those chemical messengers.

That's why something so simple creates such profound changes. You're not just managing symptoms–you're updating the source code.

The Evidence Is Overwhelming

I could fill this entire book with research studies. There are over 300 studies on Tapping to this date. But here are the highlights that should make even the biggest skeptic pause:

- **Cortisol Reduction:** Multiple studies show Tapping reduces cortisol (the primary stress hormone) 24 to 43 percent in a single session. Comparatively, talk therapy shows about 14 percent reduction in the same timeframe.[1]
- **Gene Expression:** A 2016 study found that one hour of Tapping positively affected the expression of 72 genes—including genes involved in inflammation reduction and immune function.[2]
- **Physiological Shifts:** A 2019 study found Tapping improved multiple physiological markers of health including blood pressure, heart rate, immune markers, and more.[3]
- **Brain Changes:** fMRI studies consistently show decreased activity in the areas related to cravings and pain after Tapping.[4]
- **Clinical Effectiveness:** Tapping has amassed enough evidence that it satisfies many of the methodological benchmarks laid out by APA Division 12 for potential designation as an "efficacious" therapy. Studies have found that effect sizes are large, results are rapid, and benefits last.[5]
- **PTSD Treatment:** One study in veterans found 90 percent of participants no longer met PTSD criteria after 6 sessions of Tapping.[6]

But you know what? You don't need to memorize these statistics. You already have the only evidence that truly matters: your own experience from 10 minutes ago.

The Revolution in Your Hands

Twenty years ago, if you told me that millions of people would be updating their nervous systems with their fingertips, I'm honestly not sure I would have believed you. I might have hoped for it, but did I think it would happen? Not necessarily.

But here we are. The research is in. The results are undeniable. And the power is literally in your hands.

You don't need:

- Expensive equipment
- Years of training
- A medical degree
- Perfect understanding of how it works

You just need to tap.

You don't need anyone else to change your wiring. You don't need permission, certification, or special circumstances. You have everything you need: your awareness, your fingertips, and the willingness to try.

Every person you'll read about in this book started exactly where you are: skeptical but curious, tired of their patterns, ready for something different.

Think about John, who ended up with severe insomnia after a major surgery. After he began tapping every night, his insomnia disappeared. His brain learned a new way to respond to bedtime.

Or Erin, who spent 17 years battling anxiety and depression, only to try Tapping and find herself feeling better than ever after just a few sessions.

Or 72-year-old Gary with his 15 years of back pain. One round of Tapping. Pain gone.

These aren't miracles. They're examples of what happens when you update old programming instead of trying to manage it.

Recognizing Your Current Loop

The first step to rewiring is recognizing the current Reactive Loop you're in. Let's identify your most common one.

Think about a typical day. When do you most often find yourself thinking, "Ugh, why do I always do this?"

And then think through each of the following. You can jot down notes if you find it helpful.

The Trigger: What happens just before you find yourself in the loop? (e.g., *My boss sent a one-word e-mail, or a car cuts me off in traffic, or my shoulder pain acts up again.*)

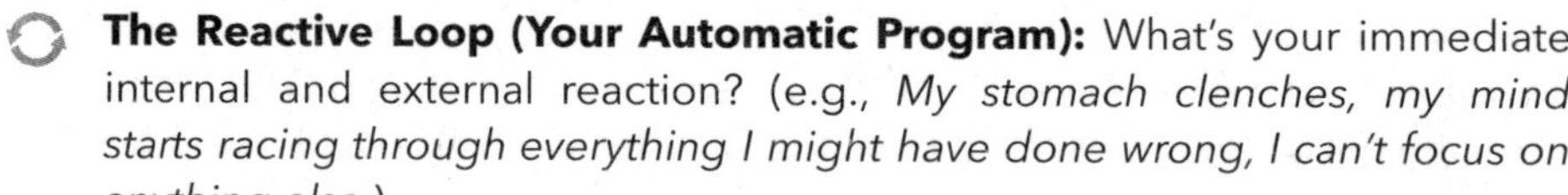

The Reactive Loop (Your Automatic Program): What's your immediate internal and external reaction? (e.g., *My stomach clenches, my mind starts racing through everything I might have done wrong, I can't focus on anything else.*)

The Cost: What does this Reactive Loop cost you? (e.g., *An hour of productivity, my peace of mind for the rest of the afternoon, my ability to be present with my family tonight.*)

Just seeing the pattern clearly is a huge step. Now you know exactly what you'll be interrupting with Tapping.

Your Next Move

You now have two things:

- A technique that takes just minutes to use
- An understanding of why it actually works

But information without action is just entertainment.

Before you read another page, I want you to start to practice recognizing. Just notice your loops. Don't judge them. Don't try to fix them. Just recognize:

"Oh, there's my worried-about-money loop."

"There's my snapping-at-my-kids pattern."

"There's my avoiding-that-task loop."

Recognition alone begins to loosen their grip. Add interruption through Tapping, and you're on your way to completely new responses.

So your mission for the next 24 hours is simple: Tap on three different Reactive Loops you notice. Anything that bothers you. Familiar stress stuck in traffic? Tap in the car. Feel annoyed at an e-mail? Tap before responding. Can't fall asleep? Tap in bed.

Each time you tap, you're not just managing that moment's stress. You're proving to your nervous system that change is possible. You're building your rewiring muscles.

In the next chapter, we'll tackle specific patterns that keep millions of us stuck, starting with the sense of overwhelm that just feels like too much. You'll learn exactly how to quiet racing thoughts and find peace in a noisy world.

But first, go tap on something. Right now. Because the more you experience this working, the more you'll trust it when we tackle the bigger stuff.

Your rewiring has begun. And it only gets better from here.

CHAPTER 4

When It All Feels Like Too Much

Finding Ground in Overwhelm

"I haven't been able to relax since . . . well ever."

That's how Jennifer, 41 years old, described her life when she first wrote to me. "I cannot get my shoulders out of my ears!"

Maybe you can relate. Your body is permanently braced for impact. Like you're constantly walking through a minefield, even when you're just walking to the kitchen. Every muscle stays tight, ready for the next crisis, the next demand, the next thing that absolutely needs your attention right now.

The cruel joke? There *is* no "next" anymore. It's just one continuous stream of Things That Need Handling. Email notifications. Text alerts. Work deadlines. Family needs. Bills. News. Social obligations. Health concerns. The dog throwing up at 5 A.M. That weird noise your car started making. The friend who's going through something and needs support. The project that was due yesterday. The appointment you forgot to schedule. The conversation you've been avoiding.

It never stops. It just . . . accumulates.

Jennifer had tried meditation many times. "But I'm too much of a busy body to sit still and do nothing physically," she explained. The very thing that everyone says should help her relax made her *more* anxious because she couldn't stop moving, couldn't stop thinking about everything else she should be doing instead of sitting there trying to breathe properly.

Then she discovered Tapping. And for the first time in 41 years, her shoulders came down.

"The tapping allows my body to move and my mind to rest," she wrote. "The perfect combination for me. I look so different with my shoulders down. lol."

I love the addition of that "lol." It sounds like genuine surprise. Like she's seeing herself clearly for the first time and realizing, "Oh. Is this what I'm supposed to look like?"

Jennifer discovered what millions are learning: that state of perpetual overwhelm—where everything feels urgent and your body never fully relaxes—isn't just a personality trait. And it certainly doesn't have to be "just how life is."

It's a Reactive Loop that can be interrupted and rewired.

HOW IS YOUR BODY FEELING RIGHT NOW?

Take a moment right now to notice your body. Where are *your* shoulders? Are there areas of your body that are tight or tense? Or do you feel relaxed and at ease?

When Stress Level 9 Becomes Your Normal

Scott was skeptical. Really skeptical.

"I was suspicious upon hearing this thing called 'Tapping,'" he admitted. The finance guy in him wanted data, evidence, proof. His wife rolled her eyes when he started. His daughters laughed outright seeing Dad tap on his face.

But the truth was that Scott was *stressed*. His stress levels had been living in the 8-to-9 range. Not during emergencies. Not during year-end reports. Just . . . Tuesday. Just normal life.

His body had forgotten what calm felt like. His nervous system didn't have a relaxation setting anymore—just varying degrees of emergency.

But Scott, despite feeling ridiculous, despite the family laughter, kept tapping. "I was fully into believing the placebo effect," Scott said, and "thus was willing to give this healing modality a shot. I felt if nothing else, the fact that I am trying, taking action to improve my way of life will in itself produce positive progress."

The finance guy's analytical brain actually helped here. He tracked his numbers. After each session, his stress dropped by one point. Just one. But when you're living at a 9, dropping to an 8 feels like finally loosening a belt that's been cinched too tight for years.

And then session by session, point by point, Scott's baseline transformed.

"I am now consistently at a 1 or even most recently 0 stress level!!! This app has been TRANSFORMATIONAL."

This is what I mean when I say your current settings aren't your permanent settings. Scott didn't become a different person. He just updated his default response from "hair on fire" to "I've got this."

Same life. Same job. Same three daughters (who hopefully no longer laugh at him tapping). Completely different nervous system response.

Every morning when Scott woke up, he hit a **Choice Point**: Fall into the familiar stress pattern—his particular Reactive Loop—or interrupt it with Tapping. For months, his brain chose door #1 automatically. But each Tapping session was him actively choosing door #2, building a new neural highway from "everything is urgent" to "I can handle this calmly."

This is the REWIRED process in action: **Recognize** (I'm at stress level 8 again), **Interrupt** (tap before the day spirals), **Rewire** (install a new baseline of calm).

And here's what's happening in your body during this process: When Scott's stress was at 8 to 9, his HPA axis (hypothalamic-pituitary-adrenal axis) was chronically activated, pumping out cortisol and adrenaline like a broken faucet. His sympathetic nervous system was stuck in the "on" position. Tapping helped flip the switch, activating his parasympathetic nervous system—the rest-and-restore mode where healing happens.

On a scale of 1 to 10, what's your baseline stress level been this week?

The Hidden Cost of Living in Emergency Mode

We are living in an age where your nervous system thinks you're being chased by bears 24/7. Except there are no bears. Just e-mails. Just traffic. Just that weird tone in your partner's voice when they asked about dinner.

Your body doesn't know the difference.

When Jennifer's shoulders lived by her ears for 41 years, her body was burning through resources like she was in active combat. When Scott operated at stress level 8 to 9 as his baseline, his system was flooding with cortisol and adrenaline meant for actual emergencies, not Tuesday afternoon meetings.

You should be getting excited right about now! Why? Because once you understand this, you realize something profound:

You're not weak. You're not failing at life. You're not "bad at handling stress."

You're having a completely normal biological response to an abnormal world.

This is part of the Great Forgetting—we've forgotten that constant stress isn't our natural state.

Your nervous system evolved for a reality where threats were clear, immediate, and temporary. Lion appears, you run. Lion gone, you relax. But modern life? It's like being stalked by an invisible lion that never quite attacks but never quite goes away either.

No wonder your shoulders are up so high, it's like they are trying to become earrings. No wonder you can't relax. No wonder you're walking around at an 8-to-9 stress level.

Your body is doing *exactly* what it's designed to do—it just doesn't realize the "danger" is an overflowing inbox, not an actual predator.

When your amygdala sounds the alarm, it isn't just raising your heart rate—it's recruiting your entire body into a survival state. Blood flow is redirected from your gut to your limbs, the vagus nerve shifts you into fight-or-flight mode, and stress hormones prime your immune cells for attack. In that moment, your brain's decision-making hub, the prefrontal cortex, temporarily powers down. Neuroscientists call this "amygdala hijack"—a short circuit where your ancient survival systems override the networks responsible for logic, memory, and empathy. In modern life, the saber-toothed tiger never shows up—but the stress cascade never shuts off.

Why This Matters More Than You Think

Here's what living in constant overwhelm is actually doing to you:

- **Your body is aging faster.** Chronic stress shortens your telomeres—the protective caps on your DNA. You're not just feeling older; stress is making you older at the cellular level.
- **Your brain is rewiring for more stress.** Remember the Familiarity Trap from Chapter 3? Every day you spend at stress level 8, your brain

gets better at being stressed. It's like training for the Anxiety Olympics when you never signed up to compete.

- **Your capacity for joy is shrinking.** When your nervous system is in constant emergency mode, it can't access states of play, creativity, or deep connection. You're surviving, not thriving.
- **Your relationships are suffering.** It's hard to be present with loved ones when your body thinks you're under attack. It's hard to be patient when you're running on emergency power.

But here's the incredible part, and why I'm so excited to share this with you:

All of this can change. Not through years of therapy. Not through quitting your job and moving to a monastery. But through a ridiculously simple technique you already learned.

THE PRICE *of* PERPETUAL EMERGENCY

What has your "perpetual emergency" stolen from you?

What have you said no to because you're already at capacity?

- ❑ That creative project gathering dust?
- ❑ The friend you keep meaning to call?
- ❑ The hobby you "don't have time for"?
- ❑ The vacation you can't take because you can't disconnect?
- ❑ The book you'll read "when things calm down"?
- ❑ The simple joy of a quiet evening at home?

Name it now. What has this cost you?

Why Tapping Works When Everything Else Failed

You've tried everything, haven't you?

The meditation apps that made you more anxious because you couldn't sit still. The breathing exercises that somehow made you more aware of how badly you were breathing. The yoga class where you spent the entire savasana mentally reorganizing your closet. The time management systems that became another source of overwhelm.

I'm as big a fan of yoga and breathwork and organization systems as anyone. I practice all these things regularly.

But sometimes they might not work the way you'd hoped, or maybe their effects don't last as long as expected. And here's why: They are asking you to be calm while your nervous system is convinced you are under attack.

It's like trying to sleep while a fire alarm is blaring. The problem isn't your sleeping technique—it's that nobody turned off the alarm.

Tapping works differently. When you tap while acknowledging your overwhelm, several things happen simultaneously:

- **Your amygdala gets confused (in the best way).** You're talking about stress while your body is receiving calming signals. Your brain goes: "Wait, she's saying she's overwhelmed, but her body is getting a massage? Maybe this isn't actually an emergency?"
- **Your cortisol drops.** Studies show Tapping reduces cortisol by up to 43 percent in a single session. That's your stress hormone draining out of your system.
- **Your nervous system shifts gears.** From sympathetic (fight-flight-freeze) to parasympathetic (rest-digest-restore). Not through forcing it, but through biological signaling that bypasses your conscious mind.
- **Your body releases.** Those shoulders that have been earrings for decades? They remember they're allowed to drop. That chest that's been tight since 2019? It remembers how to expand.

This is what happened to Jennifer from earlier. After 41 years—41 YEARS—of shoulders by her ears, a few rounds of Tapping, and they dropped.

Remember what she said? "I look so different with my shoulders down. lol."

That "lol" gets me every time. :)

The Birthday Party Reset

Let me tell you about the day I almost missed being present for my sister's birthday—not because *I* almost didn't make it, but because my nervous system almost got stuck at home with a screaming toddler.

It was one of those perfect summer afternoons. Ellis, my three-year-old, was playing outside. I had some time to spare before heading to my sister's birthday party, a big family celebration I'd been looking forward to for weeks.

Then Ellis dropped the pool skimmer on his toes.

What followed was two hours of the kind of screaming only a hurt, overtired toddler can produce. The kind that drills into your skull and activates every parental alarm bell in your system. I checked his toes (they were bloody, but after a few bandages, they were healing up just fine), tried every soothing technique in my arsenal (which was proving useless), and eventually just held him while he wailed.

By the time I left for the party, the stress had gotten to me. My jaw was clenched. My nervous system was convinced we were still in crisis mode, even though Ellis had finally calmed down and was safe.

I could have shown up to that party in body but not in spirit—stressed, distracted, still hearing phantom toddler screams. How many celebrations have we all attended while our nervous systems were stuck somewhere else?

I hit a **Choice Point**. Door #1: Show up stressed, miss my sister's joy, let Ellis's meltdown steal another moment. Door #2: Do five minutes of Tapping to remind my system that the crisis had passed.

I could show up to that party stuck in my Reactive Loop—stressed, distracted, hearing phantom toddler screams. Or I could interrupt the pattern and rewire my response.

The Familiarity Trap wanted me to stay stressed (that's what "responsible parents" do, right?). But I had a tool to help me at my fingertips. Something I could use right then and there.

So in the car, still hearing the echo of Ellis's cries, I tapped. Nothing fancy. No special words. Just tapping to remind my body that all was okay now.

Five minutes. That's all.

By the time I walked into my sister's party, I was actually there. Present. Laughing. Able to celebrate instead of just going through the motions. My nervous system had gotten the memo: Crisis over. You can enjoy your life now.

This is what I mean when I say Tapping isn't just for the big life stressors or the life overhauls. It's for life. It's for the Tuesday afternoon when your kid melts down, but you still want to show up for the people you love. It's for shifting from emergency mode to enjoyment mode, even when the echo of stress is still ringing in your ears.

The Science That Should Have You Calling Everyone You Know

Lindsey's story gives us hard data on what's happening here.

Her chiropractor had been measuring her nervous system function for two years using HRV (heart-rate variability) technology. HRV measures the variation between heartbeats; a higher variation means your nervous system is more flexible and resilient. Think of it like a stress-o-meter for your nervous system. Despite regular adjustments, Lindsey's scores stayed stuck—her system locked in fight-or-flight mode.

Then she did something different. For 90 days, she started each morning with Tapping. Just one "Create a Great Day" session. For only about five minutes.

When she went back for testing? Her HRV had jumped from 66 to 77 (that's a *big* jump for HRV; it's not that common to see a change that big, that quickly). Her nervous system had shifted from chronic emergency mode toward optimal function. The chiropractor wanted to know exactly what she'd been doing.

"Tapping," she told him. "Just Tapping."

This isn't the placebo effect at work. It certainly isn't just positive or wishful thinking. What Lindsey experienced was a measurable, biological change in how her nervous system operates.

She had systematically retrained her nervous system's baseline. By interrupting her morning stress pattern with Tapping, she actually increased her body's capacity to handle life's demands.

And remember: Lindsey was pregnant during this time. If a pregnant woman dealing with all that comes with growing a human can shift her nervous system that dramatically in 90 days, what's possible for you?

The Compound Effect Nobody Talks About

Here's something nobody tells you about rewiring your stress response: You don't just go from stressed to calm. You go from stressed to capable. From overwhelmed to overflow—having more than enough energy, clarity, and presence for whatever life brings.

When your nervous system isn't in constant emergency mode, something remarkable happens. You don't just manage better—you actually become more capable. Your decision making improves because your prefrontal cortex is back online. Creative solutions appear because your brain isn't tunnel-visioned on survival. Your energy increases because you're not burning it all on false alarms.

Scott from earlier—the one who went from an 8 or 9 on the stress scale to a 0 or 1? He didn't just feel less stressed. He became a better dad, a better employee, a better version of himself. Not through trying harder, but through rewiring his stress response.

The goal isn't to have less to handle. It's to expand your capacity to handle life gracefully, and without depleting yourself.

Moving from Overwhelm Paralysis to Simple Action

My brother, Alex, once told me: "If there's one emotion that has prevented me from taking action more than any other, it's overwhelm."

But once he realized that overwhelm was just his nervous system's panic response to "too much," everything changed.

He learned this lesson the hard way, during a period when our work was exploding, life was demanding, and everything felt urgent. The more overwhelmed he felt, the more stuck he became. It was like being paralyzed by too many options, too many priorities, too many fires to put out.

Is any part of you nodding along right now? Have you ever experienced that state where you have so much to do that you end up doing nothing? Where the sheer volume of demands makes you want to crawl back into bed?

Here's the secret Alex has since learned. When you feel that familiar paralysis creeping in (a common Familiarity Trap), don't try to just push through. Don't make another list or try a new productivity system. Instead, stop and tap on the sense of overwhelm itself.

Five minutes. That's usually all it takes to go from "I can't do anything" to "Okay, what's actually the next small step?"

Because here's the secret: When you clear the overwhelm, you discover that life isn't actually built on managing everything perfectly. It's built on small, daily actions. And you can't take those actions when your nervous system is in full panic mode about everything you haven't done yet.

"Success isn't about doing the right thing all the time," Alex explains. "It's about doing things and showing up more often than not. But you can't show up when you're paralyzed by overwhelm."

The most successful people he knows aren't the ones who never feel overwhelmed. They're the ones who've learned to clear it quickly when it arises. They fail more than others because they simply take action and try more than others.

So the next time you feel that crushing weight of too much to do, remember: The solution isn't to figure out how to do it all. It's to tap away the overwhelm so you can see clearly enough to take just one small step. Then another. Then another.

Because that's how a beautiful life actually gets built. One small action at a time.

Courtroom Calm: When Resilience Becomes Your New Normal

Jasna works in the court system in Croatia. If you want a masterclass in human stress, spend a day in any courthouse—the conflict, the high stakes, the emotional intensity. Now imagine that being your daily environment.

After starting a daily morning Tapping practice, Jasna noticed something her colleagues couldn't miss: She was the calm in their storm. They began asking what had changed. "I always tell them it's the Tapping," she said.

"Things that used to stress me out completely don't affect me the same way anymore," Jasna told me. But here's what's remarkable—her job didn't get easier. The cases didn't become less intense. The system didn't become less demanding.

She became resilient.

But the real test came during a perfect storm of crisis. A major earthquake hit during COVID. Imagine the ground literally shaking beneath you while the world was already falling apart.

"You're obviously still shaken from an earthquake," Jasna explained, "but Tapping helped me feel settled and safe and able to think clearly."

Her transformation was so obvious that even her skeptical husband couldn't ignore it. He wasn't "into this kind of stuff," but during COVID, the news was overwhelming him. The man who was so skeptical at his wife's Tapping finally asked her to show him how.

Five days. That's all it took.

After five days, his relationship with the news completely changed. There was now a protective wall between him and the news. He could watch it and not be as activated.

As he explained it: "I can live in this world and hear the news and not be as triggered." This is the compound effect in action. It's not about avoiding stress or creating a life without challenges. It's about changing your nervous system's setpoint so fundamentally that the same triggers create different, Rewired Responses.

Jasna didn't quit her stressful job. Her husband didn't stop watching the news. They didn't move to a monastery or take up permanent residence in a yoga retreat.

They stayed in their lives—earthquake, pandemic, courthouse stress, and all—but they changed their wiring. And when you change your wiring, you don't just feel better in the moment. You become someone who responds differently to life itself.

THE SOVEREIGNTY PRINCIPLE

The common thread through Jasna's, Scott's, and Jennifer's stories is a profound shift in focus. They stopped trying to make the world less stressful and instead learned to make their internal systems more resilient. They realized they couldn't control the courtroom, the economy, or the news, but they could control their response.

This is perhaps the single most powerful mindset shift you can make, a rule I call the **Sovereignty Principle.**

THE RULE:
Stop managing the world;
start regulating your nervous system.

We exhaust ourselves trying to control external variables–other people's behavior, our boss's mood, the news cycle–in a futile attempt to feel safe internally. True power, true sovereignty, lies in cultivating internal safety regardless of the external chaos.

Think of it this way: **You cannot control the waves, but you can learn to surf.** When you find yourself getting overwhelmed by things you can't control, pause and use Tapping to regulate your internal state instead. That is where your real power lies.

Your Personal Overwhelm Style

Before we tap, let's get specific about how overwhelm shows up for you. After analyzing millions of sessions, we've identified five distinct patterns. Each of these five overwhelm styles represents a specific type of Reactive Loop your nervous system has learned. Understanding your specific Overwhelm Style makes rewiring much more effective.

The Human Alarm System: Everything registers as urgent. E-mail notification? Emergency. Text message? Crisis. Someone needs something? Five-alarm fire. Your nervous system has lost the ability to distinguish between actual emergencies and normal daily life.

The Plate Spinner: You're trying to keep 17 plates spinning at once, terrified that if you stop for even a moment, everything will crash. You've become a master juggler, but you're exhausted from the constant motion.

The Yes Machine: Your overwhelm comes from saying yes when you mean no. Your calendar is full of obligations you don't want but felt you couldn't refuse. Each yes adds another weight to your already overloaded system.

The Future Borrower: You're not just dealing with today's demands—you're pre-living next week's challenges, next month's deadlines, next year's potential problems. Your nervous system is responding to stress that hasn't even happened yet.

The Absorber: You don't just handle your own stress—you soak up everyone else's too. After conversations with certain people, you feel drained, even though they were talking about their problems, not yours.

Which style resonates most? Maybe several? That's normal—overwhelm is creative in how it keeps us stuck.

Notice how each pattern is just a different flavor of the same thing? They're all variations of your nervous system forgetting how to downshift. Like a car stuck in fifth gear trying to navigate a parking lot.

The Familiarity Trap keeps you there because stressed feels safer than calm. Your brain knows stressed. It's good at stressed. Calm feels . . . suspicious. Foreign. Like something might sneak up on you if you actually relax.

PAUSE *and* REFLECT

You've read the five overwhelm styles: the Human Alarm System, the Plate Spinner, the Yes Machine, the Future Borrower, and the Absorber. Take a moment now to pause and reflect. You can write down any notes if it feels helpful.

- **Identify Your Primary Style:** Which one made you say, "Ouch, that's me"? It's okay if you're a mix, but which one or two feel most dominant?
- **Imagine the Alternative:** What would it feel like to live one day without this pattern running the show? Who would you be if your shoulders weren't by your ears? What would you do with that reclaimed energy?

The Woman with Relaxed Shoulders

As we close this chapter, I want you to imagine something:

Looking in the mirror and seeing shoulders where they belong—not up by your ears, not braced for impact, just . . . relaxed. Resting. Like they trust that you can handle whatever comes without pre-tensing for disaster.

Checking your phone without your chest tightening.
Reading your to-do list without feeling like you're drowning.
Moving through a full day and still having energy left at the end.
Having the same full life but feeling spacious instead of stuffed.

This isn't fantasy. This is what Jennifer, Scott, Jasna, and Lindsey discovered. Not a life with fewer responsibilities, but a nervous system that doesn't treat every responsibility like a five-alarm fire.

Every time you tap when overwhelmed, you're teaching your body a new truth: You can handle life without being in constant emergency mode. You can be busy without being buried. You can care without carrying the world on those (finally relaxed) shoulders.

Jennifer lives this now. Scott lives this now. Thousands of people who've tapped their way from emergency mode to easy mode live this now.

And they all started exactly where you are: skeptical, exhausted, wondering if anything could really change.

Your stress doesn't need to live at an 8. Your shoulders don't need to be earrings. Your nervous system doesn't need a constant IV drip of adrenaline.

The calm, capable version of you isn't a myth. It's just been buried under layers of false alarms and emergency broadcasts. Each tap clears some static. Each session teaches your system: We're safe. We can handle this. We can even thrive.

Ready to find out what life feels like when everything doesn't feel like too much? Ready to find out what you look like with relaxed shoulders?

Let's tap.

RECLAIMING *Your* FREEDOMS

The pattern we explored in this chapter doesn't just cause discomfort; it actively steals some of your 7 Freedoms. By using Tapping to rewire this pattern, you're not just getting rid of a problem—you're reclaiming your birthright to a full, vibrant life.

Take a moment to reflect: Which of these freedoms would open up the most for you if this pattern no longer had a hold on you?

- The freedom to experience emotions without being overwelmed.
- The freedom to respond with wisdom instead of reacting from old wounds.
- The freedom to feel calm in situations that used to throw you.
- The freedom to access energy you didn't know you had.
- The freedom to feel at home and peaceful in your body.
- The freedom to trust yourself to handle whatever comes your way.
- The freedom to show up as your real self, not who you've been conditioned to be.

What is the first thing you would do, create, or experience with this newfound freedom?

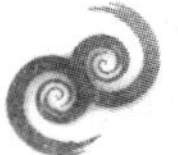

TAPPING SCRIPT: *From Overwhelm to Calm*

Let's start by checking in.

How stressed or overwhelmed are you feeling right now? Just notice where you are in this moment. Give it a number from 0 to 10, where 10 is "everything feels completely overwhelming" and 0 is you feel at ease.

Take a gentle breath in . . . and out.

Start tapping on the side of your hand. Repeat either in your mind or out loud.

When It All Feels Like Too Much

Side of the Hand: Even though I feel all this stress,
I acknowledge how I feel.

Even though there's so much going on,
and it can feel like too much,
I give myself permission to pause in this moment.

Even though I feel this tension in my body,
I choose to be gentle with myself.

Eyebrow: All this stress
Side of the Eye: All this tension
Under the Eye: This familiar feeling of overwhelm
Under the Nose: It feels like too much
Under the Mouth: There's always something to deal with
Collarbone: It's exhausting
Under the Arm: I don't even know where to start
Top of the Head: It feels hard to truly relax

Eyebrow: What if I could pause right here?
Side of the Eye: Just for this moment
Under the Eye: Nothing needs fixing right now
Under the Nose: It is safe to slow down
Under the Mouth: Even if my circumstances don't change,
Collarbone: I have more power than I realize
Under the Arm: Even in the middle of everything,
Top of the Head: I can still find some ease

Eyebrow: I give myself more credit . . .
Side of the Eye: for how far I've come . . .
Under the Eye: and for how much I've grown
Under the Nose: I don't need to hold on to this stress . . .
Under the Mouth: to get things done
Collarbone: I am ready to embrace more ease . . .
Under the Arm: and find a new way to move forward
Top of the Head: I can be peacefully productive

Eyebrow:	I am capable and strong
Side of the Eye:	I can handle whatever comes next
Under the Eye:	For now, I give myself a break
Under the Nose:	Breathing a little more deeply
Under the Mouth:	Softening my body a little more
Collarbone:	Feeling grounded in this moment
Under the Arm:	Giving myself this reassurance
Top of the Head:	I am safe and okay

Gently stop tapping and let your hands rest. Take a deep breath in . . . and let it out slowly.

Check back in with yourself now. Where's your stress level on that 0-to-10 scale? Even a small shift is your nervous system learning that you can interrupt the stress pattern.

You've just created a pocket of calm in the middle of your day. Remember, you can return here anytime you need a reset.

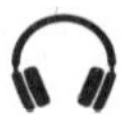

For a guided audio version of this Tapping meditation, visit www.thetappingsolution.com/rewired.

To Remember . . .

The Core Insight: *The hopeful truth is that your overwhelm is not a personal failing; it is a changeable biological pattern. Your nervous system is stuck in an emergency pattern, but you have the power to interrupt it. The world will never be less demanding. Your power lies not in managing the million things outside of you, but in mastering the one thing you can: your own internal state.*

The Practice: *See the first signs of stress—the tight shoulders, the shallow breath—as your cue to act. It's your body asking for a moment of safety. Your practice is not to push through the chaos, but to pause within it. This is a conscious act of agency, teaching your body, one moment at a time, that it has a choice other than to sound the alarm.*

CHAPTER 5

When Your Mind Won't Shut Up

Quieting the Mental Storm

Your brain comes with a special feature nobody ordered: 24/7 director's commentary on your life.

Not the fun kind where filmmakers share behind-the-scenes insights. No, this is more like having a hyperactive critic providing real-time analysis of everything you do, say, or think about doing or saying. And nobody asked for it.

"Hey, remember that thing you said in 2007? Let's analyze it from seventeen different angles."

"Speaking of analysis, here's everything that could go wrong tomorrow. And next week. And in 2035."

"Oh, and while we're here, let's replay that awkward conversation from this afternoon. We're going to analyze it in every single detail possible. Frame by frame."

Welcome to life with a mind that won't shut up.

The cruel irony? The more you try to stop thinking, the louder your thoughts get. When you're stuck in a mental spin cycle, this particular Reactive Loop of overthinking, your sympathetic nervous system interprets your efforts to "stop thinking" as even more threat. It's like telling yourself not to think about pink elephants—suddenly your mind is a Pink Elephant Convention with special guest appearances by Purple Giraffes and Neon Zebras.

"Just stop thinking," you tell yourself, which is about as effective as telling a waterfall to stop falling.

THE QUICKSAND RULE

This experience is so universal, it deserves its own law of physics for the nervous system. I call it the Quicksand Rule.

THE RULE:
When dealing with the nervous system,
the harder you fight, the deeper you sink.

Willpower, force, and "trying harder" to silence your mind all activate the sympathetic nervous system (fight-or-flight). This is the biological opposite of the calm, parasympathetic state required for your mind to settle.

You can't *force* yourself to relax for the same reason you can't fight your way out of quicksand. The only way out is to stop struggling. Tapping is how you signal to your body that it's safe to stop fighting the mental quicksand.

The Overactive Mind That Won't Let You Truly Rest

A mind that won't shut up is, to put it mildly, exhausting.

And yet that overactive mind is the very thing that prevents you from ever being able to sit still and actually rest. For real.

When the demands of your day finally pause—maybe on your lunch break, or when you arrive home after running errands, or when you relax on the couch after dinner, or when you finally get in bed—your mind starts running laps.

Maybe it starts replaying that comment you made in the meeting that didn't land quite right. Or maybe it is racing through tomorrow's to-do list, adding items you suddenly remember with a jolt of adrenaline. Or perhaps it's spinning out elaborate worst-case scenarios about that thing your teenager said—or didn't say—at dinner.

That mental spin cycle, the one that powers up precisely when you need to power down, is a universal human experience, one that has deep roots in your nervous system and brain chemistry.

When you're caught in this mental spin cycle, your brain gets stuck in problem-solving mode, burning glucose and generating stress hormones even when there's no actual problem to solve.

But, as with every Reactive Loop, it's a pattern that can be interrupted and changed into a Rewired Response.

That committee meeting in your head? You can adjourn it. Those thoughts that play on repeat like a broken record? You can change the track. That mind that won't shut up? It's just stuck in a Reactive Loop that can be fundamentally rewired to a Rewired Response.

What's the most recent thing you've found yourself ruminating on lately? Is there something on your mind just can't let go of, where you're having the same thoughts over and over again? How would it feel if you could stop the cycle and let go of thinking about that thing?

The Ancient Fable of the Monkey Mind

There's an old Buddhist tale about a monkey trapped in a house. Desperate to escape, it races from room to room, window to window, creating chaos everywhere it goes. The more frantically it searches for an exit, the more damage it causes.

A wise teacher enters and, instead of chasing the monkey, simply opens all the windows and sits quietly in the center of the room. The monkey, no longer feeling trapped, calms down. Eventually, it finds its own way out.

Your racing thoughts? They're that monkey. And you've been chasing them from room to room, exhausting yourself while they just get more frantic.

What if, instead of chasing, you could just open the windows?

The Woman Who Fired Her Mental News Anchor

Joyce was 70 years old when she finally realized that a lifetime of sensitivity and unprocessed emotions were catching up to her.

"I started having panic attacks a few years ago, but I didn't know what they were," Joyce told us. Picture this: Seven decades of unprocessed emotions suddenly demanding attention, like a storage unit that's been sealed since 1950 suddenly bursting open. She started anti-anxiety medication and saw a therapist, but the anxiety was intense. And it affected her on a daily basis.

Her therapist introduced her to Tapping during their weekly sessions. But here's where Joyce did something brilliant—she recognized that one hour a week of relief wasn't enough when her mind was broadcasting anxiety 168 hours a week.

"I realized that neither the weekly visits nor the weekly Tapping was gonna be enough for me," she said. So Joyce did what any sensible person would do when faced with a 24/7 problem—she found a 24/7 solution.

She started tapping every single day.

Not some days. Not when she remembered. Every. Single. Day.

"I have tapped daily for 700 days," she wrote to us. "I'll be tapping the rest of my life."

Seven hundred days. A daily habit like brushing your teeth, except for your thoughts.

The result? "I no longer take any medication for anxiety. I've learned so much about my emotions and how to deal with them. It has saved my life, not joking, not exaggerating."

Remarkable, isn't it?

Every day, she hit the same **Choice Point**: spiral into panic or reach for a new response. Seven hundred times, she chose to interrupt the pattern. Seven hundred times, she proved to her nervous system: "We don't have to be who we've always been."

At 70, Joyce discovered what some people never learn: Your mental news anchor can be fired. The 24/7 broadcast can be canceled. The monkey can find the open window. It just takes a little training.

And I'm not saying it will take 700 Tapping sessions for you to notice a difference. Maybe it will take 7. Or maybe it will take 7,000. The point is that Joyce committed to doing something different for herself. To interrupt her pattern and retrain her brain for something new.

Think about how much we (rightfully) praise and celebrate people who run marathons. They commit to something, and then they train and train and train until they are able to accomplish an amazing feat.

What if we took the same approach with our mental training? What if we committed and trained and stuck with it like Joyce did?

CHOICE POINT CHECKPOINT: THE ANXIETY CROSSROADS

Every anxious moment offers the same Choice Point:

Door #1: Feed the Loop
(research symptoms, rehearse conversations, plan for disasters, etc.)

Door #2: Interrupt with Tapping

The Familiarity Trap whispers: "But worrying keeps you safe! What if you miss something important?"

The Truth: In 20 years of Tapping, no one has ever said, "I really miss my anxiety. Life was better when I worried constantly."

So keep an eye out and notice your next anxiety Choice Point. You'll know it by the urge to reread that text for the 15th time, mentally rehearse a conversation that hasn't happened yet, think about all possible scenarios, or Google information till the sun goes down.

That's your cue to Recognize, Interrupt, Rewire.

The Biology Behind the Buzz

Have you ever wondered why your mind races most intensely right when you're trying to relax? Or why logical reassurance ("I know everything will be fine") does absolutely nothing to shut down those racing, repetitive thoughts?

Here's the truth bomb: Your racing mind isn't broken. It's not trying to ruin your life. It's just a little confused and misguided in its efforts to keep you safe.

It's a predictable result of an overactive amygdala sending constant "threat detected" signals to your anterior cingulate cortex (ACC), the brain region involved in attention and emotion regulation.

This creates a feedback loop: perceived threat → increased vigilance → scanning for more threats → finding them (because you're looking) → reinforcing the original threat perception.

Think of it like a guard dog that barks at leaves, clouds, and suspicious-looking shadows. Super dedicated. Terrible at threat assessment. Kind of like my mini bernedoodle puppy Willow, who has a hard time with shadows at night when I take her out to use the bathroom.

You don't need to get rid of the guard dog. You just need to teach it the difference between "actual burglar" and "wind moving the curtains."

When your mind won't shut up, what's really happening is your nervous system is locked in a biological stress response. Your amygdala—essentially your brain's smoke detector—has been triggered, and it's not just making noise. It's firing signals to your hypothalamus, which flips on your body's stress switch. The hypothalamus then activates the autonomic nervous system and the HPA axis (hypothalamic-pituitary-adrenal), setting off a whole-body cascade: Your adrenal glands pump out adrenaline and cortisol, your heart races, your breathing quickens, digestion slows, and blood is shunted to your muscles in case you need to run or fight.

The catch? Unlike a real smoke detector that goes quiet when the air clears, your brain's alarm can keep ringing long after the "smoke" is gone. Elevated cortisol keeps the system humming, your muscles stay tense, your stomach stays unsettled, and your thoughts keep circling—like an engine that won't turn off. This is why you can't "think" your way out of overthinking. In fact, trying to logic your way out just feeds the loop—it's like trying to put out a fire by throwing matches on it.

The Invisible Thief in Your Head

That mental spin cycle, that particular type of Reactive Loop where thoughts replay endlessly, feels like a private, internal problem. But it's robbing you blind in the real world, stealing the very things that make life worth living.

Why should you care about taming this "director's commentary"? Because its impact goes far beyond your own skull:

- **It steals your presence.** You were physically there when your daughter told you about her day, but were you *really* there? Or were you mentally rehearsing tomorrow's meeting? Your racing mind costs you the irreplaceable moments of your actual life.
- **It compromises your health.** The constant "what-if" replay keeps your body in a low-grade stress response, contributing to everything from insomnia and digestive issues to tension headaches and a weakened immune system. Your thoughts are just adding to your body's struggle.

- **It hijacks your identity.** After years of this pattern, you stop saying, "I'm having anxious thoughts" and start saying, "I am an anxious person." The pattern becomes your identity, limiting what you believe is possible for yourself.

This chapter isn't about achieving some impossible state of Zen-like inner peace. It's about saying "no more" to the thief who has been living in your head, stealing your peace, your presence, and your health.

It's about discovering who you are and how you feel when your mind is a little bit calmer and little bit quieter—not an incessant chatter of all the worrisome things.

THE MOMENTS YOU'RE MISSING

While your mind is having its board meeting at the least convenient times, what are you actually missing?

- ❑ Your partner talking about their day (while you nod on autopilot)
- ❑ Your kid's story (while you mentally write e-mails)
- ❑ The movie you're "watching" (while solving tomorrow's problems)
- ❑ The meal you're eating (while your brain is elsewhere)
- ❑ This moment, right now (while thinking about the next one)

Actually pause and reflect on that for a moment. What is this costing you?

Your life is happening while you're busy thinking about your life.

The Overthinking Olympics: Which Event Are You Training For?

I've worked with thousands of people whose minds won't shut up, and I've noticed something that would be funny if it wasn't so costly: We all specialize. Like athletes who excel at different events, we each have our signature style of mental overdrive. It's like the Olympics of overthinking.

Which kind of mental "athlete" are you?

Event #1: Mental Time Travel

You're a world-class mental archaeologist, digging up conversations from 1997 and examining them with the dedication of someone searching for ancient treasure. Except instead of gold, you find embarrassment, shame, sadness, disappointment, regret . . . Every. Single. Time.

You're constantly shuttling between past regrets and future disasters, never stopping in the present where, ironically, everything is usually fine. Your brain treats time like a playground where all the equipment is made of anxiety.

Have you ever replayed a moment so many times it feels more real than the present?

Have you caught yourself stressing about something that already happened—or hasn't happened yet?

Event #2: Catastrophe Forecasting

You've turned worry into an art form. Give you any situation, and you'll transform it into a five-act tragedy before breakfast. A child's cough becomes pneumonia. A boss's "we need to talk" becomes unemployment. Your brain's motto: "But what if . . . ?"

Your imagination deserves recognition for "Most Creative Disaster Scenarios." While others see a delayed text response, you see relationship doom. While they see traffic, you see inevitable lateness leading to job loss leading to financial ruin.

Have you ever taken one tiny worry and turned it into a full-blown disaster?

Have you noticed how often you assume the worst-case scenario, even though it almost never actually ends up happening?

Event #3: The Self-Prosecution Trial

You run a 24/7 courtroom in your head where you're always the defendant and somehow also the harshest judge.

Every mistake becomes a new charge. Every success is dismissed as luck. Your inner prosecutor has never lost a case because the verdict is always the same: guilty of not being good enough.

Do you ever judge yourself harshly for something you'd easily forgive in a friend?

Have you ever let a single mistake define your whole self-worth?

Event #4: Analysis Paralysis

You approach every interaction like it's an ancient text requiring translation. That "hmm" from your partner launches a full investigation. Was it disappointed? Contemplative? Passive-aggressive? Time to analyze tone, duration, and historical "hmm" patterns.

E-mail composition becomes your marathon event. "Should I say 'Best' or 'Sincerely'? Is the exclamation point too aggressive? What if they misinterpret my tone?" Three hours later, you've written two sentences and created 17 drafts.

Have you ever spent 20 minutes rereading one text before hitting Send?

Have you wasted so much time deciding that the moment passed anyway?

Event #5: The Comparison Championships

Your specialty is comparing your behind-the-scenes footage to everyone else's highlight reel—and always losing. You're convinced others received the "Life Instructions Manual" while you're desperately improvising.

Your midnight research confirms it: They sleep better. Worry less. Have functional brains with actual off switches. You've studied their social media, analyzed their apparent ease, and concluded you're uniquely defective.

In this event, the rules ensure you never win. Their success is talent; yours is luck. Their struggles are temporary; yours are permanent. Your mental scoreboard always shows you in last place.

Have you scrolled social media and suddenly felt like your whole life was off track?

Have you ever believed everyone else has it figured out but you?

Which Event Is *Your* Specialty?

Really pause and consider that for a moment. Get to know your inner chatter a bit better.

Maybe you've perfected one particular discipline, training unconsciously for years in your signature event. Or maybe you find yourself trying to compete in all of them simultaneously.

Each of these events is a **Familiarity Trap** in action. Your brain has gotten so good at Mental Time Travel or Catastrophe Forecasting that it feels safer to keep competing than to try something new.

Even though these mental Olympics are exhausting, they're familiar. And to your nervous system, familiar equals safe—even when it's making you miserable.

But here's what every mental Olympian needs to know: These aren't permanent assignments.

It's not that you need to become a better competitor.

You need to realize something: You can withdraw from the games entirely.

So, are you ready to hand in your uniform?

The Math Nobody Teaches You

Here's an equation that should be taught in schools:

Racing Thoughts + Fighting Them = Thoughts x 100

The more you wrestle with your thoughts, the stronger they get. It's like trying to smooth out water by slapping it—you just make more waves.

But here's the equation that changes everything:

Racing Thoughts + Tapping = Thoughts ÷ 100 (or more)

And we have the data to prove it. After 1.7 million plays of our "Release Anxiety" session, users report an average 40 percent reduction in anxiety in just 9 minutes.

Study upon study back this up. One study found an average reduction in anxiety of 58 percent.[7] A meta-analysis of 14 studies with 658 participants found that Tapping produced a massive effect size (Cohen's d = 1.23) for anxiety reduction.[8] To put that in perspective, anything above 0.8 is considered a "large" effect. Tapping blew past that benchmark.

And speed? While traditional therapy might take 8 to 12 weekly sessions to produce noticeable anxiety reduction, many Tapping studies achieved similar or better results in just 2 to 4 sessions.

The 20-Year-Old and the Midnight Miracle

Addie was 20 and thought anxiety was something that happened to other people. You know, anxious people. Not her.

Then a side effect from a new medication for another health issue hit her like a surprise party nobody wanted. "My life turned for the worst. I quit the medication after a week, but my life still consisted of feeling anxious 24/7."

Picture being 20 years old and suddenly your brain won't stop throwing its own rave. Except instead of music, it's playing your worst fears on repeat. "I couldn't eat, sleep, go to class, hang out with friends, or even take care of my hygiene. I was in a never-ending cycle of just getting through the day."

Her mind raced constantly—during lectures, while trying to spend time with friends, even during what should have been relaxing Netflix sessions. The simplest activities became marathons of mental endurance.

Then her therapist did something unexpected. In the middle of their session, he pulled out his phone to show her something he'd logged over 100 minutes on. "He told me it changed his life."

Addie thought, "How can tapping on my hand get rid of these uncontrollable feelings?"

Fair question. But that night, desperate, she tried it. And then this happened:

"About twenty minutes ago, I felt a panic attack come on at 12 A.M. I felt my body tense up and my mind race, so I opened my app and begun a breathing and Tapping exercise. Afterwards, I felt so much better that I decided to answer your e-mail about how much Tapping has helped me in the middle of the night!"

She went from panic attack to writing thank-you e-mails. At midnight. That's like going from hurricane to gentle breeze in the time it takes to microwave popcorn.

"I'll never understand the science behind Tapping," Addie admitted, "but I'm so grateful I was recommended it. My anxiety still lingers, but I wouldn't be where I am if it wasn't for my therapist telling me about Tapping!"

The Plot Twist Nobody Expects

Here's what people discover that shocks them every time:

You don't have to stop your thoughts to find peace.

You don't have to achieve monk-like mental silence. You don't have to win a battle against your own brain. You don't have to become someone you're not.

You just have to change the relationship with your mind.

It's like living with a roommate who plays music too loud. You don't need to evict them or destroy the stereo. You just need to address the issue and find the volume knob.

Joyce found it after 70 years. Addie found it at 20.

They both discovered the same thing: The volume of worried thoughts can turn down. They can stop playing on repeat. And when we change how we relate to them, they no longer get to run the show.

THE MENTAL NOISE AUDIT

Let's get specific about what *your* mental noise pattern is like. You can write down your answers to these questions or simply reflect on each one.

1. **Prime Time:** When does your mind get loudest? (Morning? 3 A.M.? Sunday nights?)
2. **The Greatest Hits:** What are the top three thoughts that play on repeat in your head?
3. **The Physical Cost:** Where do you feel these racing thoughts in your body? Chest? Head? Stomach?
4. **The Possibilities Ahead:** If your mind suddenly went quiet for 24 hours, what would you finally be able to focus on? If those top three thoughts could finally stop playing, what could you use the leftover mental energy on?

What Life Looks Like After the Thoughts Lose Their Grip

"I forgot what it feels like to not have my thoughts screaming at me all the time."

That's a common realization after people start tapping regularly. Many have lived with racing thoughts for so long they've gone through a Great Forgetting and can't remember what mental quiet feels like.

So what actually happens when people break free from chronic overthinking through Tapping? Through our research with hundreds of thousands of users, we've identified several profound shifts:

The Return of Presence

The most immediate change people report is actually being where they are. Having the TV on and actually paying attention to what's on the screen. Having dinner and actually tasting the food. Listening to their kids talk and actually hearing the stories, not their own mental commentary.

Emotional Regulation Returns

When thoughts constantly trigger stress responses, emotions become reactive and volatile. As the thought patterns quiet down, emotional stability returns.

The Body Relaxes

The connection between overthinking and physical symptoms is undeniable. Chronic thought spirals trigger stress responses that manifest as headaches, digestive issues, muscle tension, and insomnia.

As one user put it: "EFT is the only practice I've ever tried over the years that makes a noticeable difference in my body every time I've used it."

Remember those cortisol reductions? That's not just numbers on a lab report. Lower cortisol means:

- Better sleep (cortisol disrupts sleep cycles)
- Improved digestion (stress hormones shut down digestive function)
- Reduced inflammation (chronic cortisol promotes inflammatory conditions)
- Stronger immunity (high cortisol suppresses immune function)

Identity Shifts

Perhaps the most surprising outcome is that people stop identifying as "overthinkers" or "anxious people."

Maybe you've always seen yourself as the "worrier" in the family. Or maybe your friends all joke about you being the overthinker of the group.

What if that didn't have to be true anymore?

RECLAIMING *Your* FREEDOMS

The pattern we explored in this chapter doesn't just cause discomfort; it actively steals some of your 7 Freedoms. By using Tapping to rewire this pattern, you're not just getting rid of a problem–you're reclaiming your birthright to a full, vibrant life.

Take a moment to reflect: Which of these freedoms would open up the most for you if this pattern no longer had a hold on you?

- The freedom to experience emotions without being overwhelmed.
- The freedom to respond with wisdom instead of reacting from old wounds.
- The freedom to feel calm in situations that used to throw you.
- The freedom to access energy you didn't know you had.
- The freedom to feel at home and peaceful in your body.
- The freedom to trust yourself to handle whatever comes your way.
- The freedom to show up as your real self, not who you've been conditioned to be.

What is the first thing you would do, create, or experience with this newfound freedom?

From Xanax to Freedom

Sharon from Georgia started her Tapping journey in an emergency room, relying on Xanax just to survive each day. Racing thoughts had hijacked her life, keeping her in constant mental motion to avoid confronting deeper pain. Her Reactive Loop had become deeply ingrained.

Tapping became a transformative tool that helped calm her body and mind in her daily life, giving her a profound sense of relief. She'd use it anywhere: even sitting in traffic. As she began to interrupt the anxious spirals running her everyday life, she was able to begin to process deeper emotions and experiences—from the unresolved anger during her divorce to deep childhood trauma.

And through Tapping, she slowly took back her life from anxiety. As she explained, she moved from dependence on medication to just make it through each day to emotional independence with the confidence to navigate even the hardest of days.

Having rewired her system for safety and calm, she was able to stay centered and strong through the unimaginable—including caring for her husband through cancer and grieving her mother after her passing.

Today, Sharon integrates Tapping with biofeedback technology as a trained technician, helping others find the same emotional freedom she discovered.

From mental chaos to mental peace. That is the journey waiting for you.

Your Invitation to Mental Peace

So here's where we are: You've been competing in the Overthinking Olympics for years, maybe decades. You've mastered every event. Your mental muscles are exhausted from the constant training.

How's that working out for you?

If you're tired of missing your actual life because you're lost in your thoughts, if you're ready to be present for the moments that matter, if you want to sit on your couch and actually relax, you're in the right place.

Because here's what we know to be true: You're not just an "anxious" or "overthinking" person. You're a person with an anxious or overthinking pattern.

You can turn down the volume. You can teach the guard dog new (and more fun) tricks. You can fire the news anchor. You can open the windows and let the monkey find its own way out.

Your racing mind has been trying to protect you. Thank it for its service. Then show it a better way.

The research is clear. The results are consistent. The tool is in your hands.

Ready to discover what your evenings feel like when you're actually there for them?

Let's tap.

TAPPING SCRIPT:
Quieting the Mental Chatter

Let's check in with your mind right now.

How busy are your thoughts? Give how you feel now a number from 0 to 10, where 10 is your thoughts feel totally overwhelming, and 0 is your mind feels quiet and at ease.

Take a gentle breath in . . . and out.

Start tapping on the side of your hand. Repeat either in your mind or out loud.

Side of the Hand: Even though my mind keeps going and going,
I acknowledge my mind's good intentions.

Even though I can't seem to turn off these thoughts,
I'm open to turning down the volume.

Even though my mind is so busy,
I choose to breathe deeply and slow down in this moment.

Eyebrow: All these thoughts
Side of the Eye: Round and round they go
Under the Eye: All this mental chatter
Under the Nose: My mind won't let me rest
Under the Mouth: Always thinking, always analyzing
Collarbone: Rarely a moment of ease
Under the Arm: It's tiring when my mind won't stop
Top of the Head: I just want a break

Eyebrow: Right now, in this moment . . .
Side of the Eye: I simply notice any thoughts
Under the Eye: I can recognize old protective patterns . . .
Under the Nose: and remind myself that I am safe
Under the Mouth: It's safe to take a break
Collarbone: I don't have to control my thoughts . . .
Under the Arm: or believe everything I think
Top of the Head: I simply become an observer

Eyebrow: Thoughts can come and go . . .
Side of the Eye: but I can stay steady and grounded
Under the Eye: There's nothing I need to figure out right now
Under the Nose: One tap at a time . . .
Under the Mouth: the volume is turning down
Collarbone: Creating a little more space . . .
Under the Arm: to tune in to myself . . .
Top of the Head: and access my own inner wisdom

Eyebrow: I get out of my head . . .
Side of the Eye: and settle back into my body
Under the Eye: I am safe to rest here
Under the Nose: Allowing my shoulders to relax
Under the Mouth: Softening my jaw
Collarbone: Releasing any remaining tension
Under the Arm: As I move throughout my day,
Top of the Head: I bring this new sense of ease with me

Gently stop tapping and let your hands rest. Take a deep breath in . . . and let it out slowly.

Notice your mind now. Rate again from 0 to 10 how overwhelming your thoughts feel right now. If you are feeling greater ease, your new number will be lower.

Great work. You've just shown your mind it's safe to slow down.

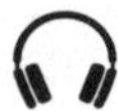
For a guided audio version of this Tapping meditation, visit www.thetappingsolution.com/rewired.

To Remember . . .

The Core Insight: *A racing mind is just a sign that your body's alarm system is active. The hopeful truth is you don't have to be a prisoner of your thoughts. Trying to fight them is like struggling in quicksand—it only makes you sink faster. The key is to stop fighting and soothe the underlying anxiety instead.*

The Practice: *Reclaim your authority. When a thought spiral begins, start tapping to remind your nervous system that you are safe. You are not trying to silence the thought; you are turning off the alarm that powers it. This is how you reclaim your mental peace.*

CHAPTER 6

When Frustration Builds

Releasing Pressure Before It Explodes

We live in an Age of Perpetual Irritation, and nobody wants to talk about it. The neighbor's leaf blower at 7 A.M. The group text that won't stop pinging. The co-worker who heats fish in the microwave. The slow walker in front of you when you're already late. The "reply all" e-mail that created chaos in the office. We're all swimming in a sea of minor frustrations that keep piling on day after day, hour after hour.

And sure, we'll admit to being "stressed" or "overwhelmed." We'll even cop to feeling worried or down. But feeling frustrated, irritated, and angry?

That's like a secret club nobody wants to admit they're in (even though we're all members).

Because angry people are "difficult." Angry people have "issues." Angry people need "anger management."

So we pretend we're fine while internally maintaining detailed mental lists of everything that frustrates us, from the person who cut in line at the grocery store last week to the uncle who can't help but bring up controversial political opinions at every single family dinner.

The membership requirements to the Secret Society of the Perpetually Frustrated are simple: Live in the modern world. Have expectations. Watch them get repeatedly crushed by reality.

And we all have our unique manifestation of this. We all have areas of life where we can hold it together and where we can't. Where we stuff it down and where it explodes out. These are our unique flavors of an angry Reactive Loop, where our nervous systems have learned to interpret everyday frustrations as threats to our survival, status, or sense of fairness.

You might be patient as a saint at work, then snap at your kids over spilled juice. Or maybe you're endlessly understanding with family, but that co-worker who interrupts you in meetings makes your blood boil over.

Helen qualified for lifetime membership as a single mom of three, two with special needs. With all the responsibilities to juggle on a daily basis, the pressure was sometimes too much to handle. She found herself snapping at her kids at even the littlest things.

Chris earned platinum status after 71 years of pent-up anger. Things from childhood, from tension in his marriage, from a conflict with his eldest daughter. It all added up to the point it couldn't help but boil over.

Sandra joined when she became caregiver to her mother, who had been emotionally distant her whole life. She felt resistant, resentful, and angry that she was left to take care of everything all on her own—on top of an already stressful day job.

Maybe you joined when your partner folded the laundry wrong for the 1,467th time. Or when your boss took credit for your best idea yet. Or when someone you trusted betrayed your confidence.

Each of these forms of frustration represents a different trigger for the same underlying Reactive Loop: the anger response. Whether it's daily irritations or systemic injustice, your nervous system runs the same biological program: threat detected → stress hormones released → prefrontal cortex offline → react from primitive brain.

The Full Spectrum of Fury

Usually, anger isn't just about one thing. It encapsulates an entire spectrum of types of frustration that color modern life in all sorts of ways.

Sometimes it's small and constant, like a stone in your shoe that isn't bad enough to fix but is noticeable with every step. And other times it's massive and overwhelming, like a tsunami that crashes over you with obvious magnitude.

Regardless, it's always there, humming in the background.

Here are a few forms of frustration that might be impacting your life:

- **The Daily Drip:** The dishwasher loaded wrong (again). The co-worker who leaves early while you stay late. The grocery store with only one checkout lane open during rush hour.
- **The Personal Wounds:** When someone you trusted cuts deep. When a family member makes that comment that hits exactly where you're most vulnerable. When someone dismisses your feelings or treats you like you don't matter.
- **The Systemic Rage:** Corporate greed while families struggle. Politicians lying with straight faces. The rigged system you can't change. This type of anger loop is particularly exhausting because your nervous system is responding to threats you genuinely can't fight or flee from. Your biology is primed for action, but there's no clear action to take.
- **The Helplessness Rage:** Your car's check engine light the same week rent increases. Running late and hitting every red light. Playing a game where the rules keep changing.

Which of these can you relate to the most? Maybe one, maybe several, maybe all?

None of these exist in isolation. They compound. They stack up. They create a constant background hum of irritation that makes everything harder than it needs to be.

And here's the kicker:

You feel guilty about feeling angry about the small stuff because "people have real problems." About the big stuff because "what can I do about it anyway?" Which just adds shame to your frustration, creating a lovely cocktail of anger and self-judgment that makes you feel even worse.

These small, constant Reactive Loops are like background programs draining your battery. The dishwasher loaded wrong triggers a micro-stress response. Your nervous system releases a squirt of cortisol. Not enough to notice, but multiply that by 50 daily irritations, and you're marinating in stress hormones.

TAKING AN HONEST ACCOUNT OF YOUR FRUSTRATION

Time for some honest accounting:

1. Name three things that consistently frustrate you (traffic, e-mails, that one co-worker, politics, etc.).
2. What percentage of your daily energy do you estimate might be going to being annoyed/frustrated/angry at those things?
3. What would open up for you if that frustration didn't consume so much of your life?

The Invisible Weight That's Eating You Alive

Let's talk about what this constant frustration and anger is actually doing to you. Because without a doubt, persistent frustration rewires your entire experience of being alive.

- **Your system is stuck in threat mode:** From household chore disputes to systemic injustice, your nervous system never gets the memo that it's safe. Stress hormones stay elevated. You're living in perpetual emergency.
- **Your relationships become collateral damage:** Loved ones get the worst of you. Partners get snapped at for breathing too loud. Kids get impatient responses.
- **Your joy gets suffocated:** Chronic frustration blocks positive experiences. Can't see the sunset—too busy fuming. Miss your child's sweet comment—mentally rehearsing that argument. Good moments happen, but you're too angry to notice.
- **Your perspective gets hijacked:** The more frustrated you get, the more frustration you find. Your brain scans for evidence that everything's unfair and everyone's incompetent. And it finds plenty, because that's what brains do—find what they're looking for.
- **Your energy leaks everywhere:** Being angry about everything is exhausting. The energy that goes to being annoyed about things leave less energy for things that matter to you.

- **Your body becomes an overworked storage facility:** Your muscles stay permanently braced for battle. Your digestive system operates in constant crisis mode. Your immune system gets confused about who the enemy is and starts attacking you instead.

Take a moment to pause and think about how frustration and anger might be showing up in your own life and in your own body. Have your relationships been taking a toll? Is your body working overtime? Is energy hard to muster these days?

Why You Can't "Just Let It Go": The Science of a Triggered Brain

We've all heard the same frustrating advice: "Just let it go." "Pick your battles." "Don't sweat the small stuff."

If you could just let it go, you would have done it already. Nobody volunteers for the constant background hum of irritation that makes everything feel harder than it should be.

Here's why that advice fails: Your frustration isn't a logical choice; it's a biological survival response. Deep in your brain, your amygdala—the alarm system we've been talking about—has been trained to interpret everything from inefficiency to injustice as a threat. Not just a physical threat, but a threat to your sense of order, fairness, and respect.

So, when your partner forgets three items on the grocery list, your amygdala doesn't register a simple mistake. It fires off a survival signal: "Threat detected! Disrespect! I can't count on them!" When a less qualified person gets the promotion over you, it registers a systemic danger: "The world is fundamentally unfair!"

Once that alarm is pulled, your body floods with stress hormones designed for a physical emergency.

Your blood pressure rises, your muscles tense, and most importantly, your prefrontal cortex, the part of your brain that provides logic, perspective, and wisdom, goes offline. This is why you literally "see red" or "can't think straight" when angry; your brain has diverted resources from thinking to fighting. You are actually having a survival response to everything from poor dishwasher technique to systemic injustice.

This is why you can feel like you're going crazy. But the reality is, you're having a normal, predictable biological reaction to what your brain perceives as an endless series of attacks on your well-being.

Every daily irritation becomes a Choice Point: fall into the familiar frustration (your Reactive Loop) or learn to interrupt the pattern at its biological source.

When Your Biggest Problem Becomes Your Biggest Block

Here's the cruel irony: The intensity of your anger often prevents you from solving the very problems you're angry about.

When you're consumed by how wrong something is, how unfair it feels, how incompetent everyone else seems to be, your brain can't access the creative, strategic thinking you need to actually shift the situation.

It's like trying to thread a needle while your hands are shaking with rage. The steadier your hands, the easier the task becomes.

My sister, Jessica, learned this the hard way when she was working on our Tapping documentary.

Tapping to Find Your Power Again

When we were working on *The Tapping Solution* documentary back in 2007, Jessica had one crucial job: get the experts from *The Secret* (such a hit at the time, and still is to this day) to agree to talk to us about Tapping.

It made perfect sense. The experts who taught the Law of Attraction often mentioned Tapping as a way to clear blocks. We figured they'd be the perfect place to start when looking for well-known professionals to include in our documentary.

The only problem was, they all said no.

One after another, the people Jessica reached out to either ignored her e-mails or politely declined. She started to feel frustrated . . . and a little bit angry.

One assistant wouldn't even share the offer with her client. It felt like such a blow to not even have the chance to get through to have a fair shot.

"I felt like such a failure," Jessica reflected later. "My one job was to get these people, and I couldn't get *anyone*. I was so frustrated. It felt like I had hit the end of the road, and I didn't have any idea what I was supposed to do next."

Jessica spent days in that familiar frustration spiral—the one where you replay every rejection, question your abilities, and convince yourself that you're not cut out for what you're trying to do.

She was stuck in what I now recognize as classic Survival Mode: her nervous system interpreting every "no" as evidence that she wasn't good enough, that the project was doomed, that she should just quit.

But then she reached a Choice Point: She could stay in the familiar frustration spiral or try something different. She chose to tap.

"I was just so frustrated," she remembers now. "I tapped on feeling like a failure, on all the rejection, on wanting to give up. And as I tapped, something shifted. My mind got quiet enough for me to actually think clearly."

Recognize: "I'm stuck in frustration, and it's blocking my thinking."

Interrupt: Instead of staying in the spiral, she tapped to break the pattern.

Rewire: With her nervous system calm, space opened up for a creative solution.

Here's what happened next: With her nervous system calm instead of hijacked by frustration, Jessica had a clear, creative thought that hadn't occurred to her before. She remembered that Joe Vitale had been in *The Secret*, but she'd never heard him talk about Tapping. What if he was into it but she just didn't know?

She looked him up. Turns out, he was deeply into Tapping.

She drove down to Austin, sat in his living room, and poured her heart out about the mission behind the documentary. Joe was so moved that he sent a personal message to Jack Canfield (a motivational speaker and co-author of the Chicken Soup for the Soul series), on Jessica's behalf.

Jack said yes. Then, like dominoes, everyone else said yes.

The entire trajectory of our documentary, and arguably our entire business, changed because Jessica tapped through her frustration instead of staying stuck in it.

The Truth About What You're Really Angry At

Here's what 20 years of helping people with chronic frustration has taught me: *You're not angry at the situation. You're angry at your powerlessness within the situation.*

When your co-worker misses the meeting you had planned, you're not really angry at the schedule mishap. You're angry that you care more about efficiency than they do. You're angry that you feel responsible for everything going smoothly on the team.

When you see injustice in the world, you're not just angry at the injustice itself. You're angry that you can't fix it. You're angry that good people suffer while bad people prosper.

When someone hurts your feelings, you're not just angry at their words. You're angry that being a good person doesn't protect you from being hurt. You're angry that you can't make people care about your feelings the way you care about theirs.

The frustration isn't about the external situation. It's about your internal desire for reality to be different than it is.

But guess what? You can change your relationship with your powerlessness. You can teach your nervous system that you're safe even when things aren't under your control. You can rewire your response to life's inevitable inefficiencies and injustices.

THE "TAP WHILE IT'S HAPPENING" RULE

This is the single most effective strategy for rewiring your reactions in real time, a non-negotiable rule I call **The "Tap While It's Happening" Mandate.**

THE RULE:
The best time to rewire a pattern is while the pattern is active.

Neuroscience shows us that a memory or emotional pattern is only changeable when it's "unlocked," meaning you are actively experiencing it. This is the golden window for what's known as memory reconsolidation. When you feel that flash of anger or the slow burn of resentment, your nervous system has just opened the file. Tapping at that exact moment allows you to edit the file before it gets saved again.

What to Do: Do not wait until later to tap on the argument, the frustrating e-mail, or the irritation. If you can, excuse yourself for 60 seconds and tap *while* you are angry. This is not about suppressing the feeling; it's about metabolizing the emotional energy on the spot so it doesn't get stored in your body. This is where the real magic happens.

The Meltdown That Could Have Gone Terribly Wrong

Greta faced a Choice Point when her seven-year-old son was having a complete meltdown at the end of an already exhausting day.

The trigger? She'd told him he couldn't play more Roblox before bed. That's when everything exploded—crying, yelling, the works.

She could have chosen the familiar frustrated Reactive Loop and escalated right along with him, which inevitably would end in a battle of the wills. Instead, she pulled her son onto her lap and tapped with him. Five minutes later, it was like a switch had gone off. All of a sudden he was calm, apologizing, coming to her for cuddles, and talking to her about what had happened.

Reflecting on the situation, he said: "I know it wasn't really such a big deal, but it felt that way when it happened."

This seven-year-old understood what most adults can't grasp: big emotions, like anger, can hijack us. But when we regulate them, we open ourselves up to a whole new perspective.

What Becomes Available When You're Not Consumed by Anger

Here's what I want to really make clear: The goal isn't to *never* feel angry.

Anger, along with frustration, irritation, and annoyance, provides important information. These emotions tell you when something violates your values, when boundaries are being crossed, when injustice is happening.

The goal is to feel your anger and release it, without being consumed by it.

Regulated anger is a superpower. It's the fuel that drives positive change without burning you out. It's the voice that speaks truth without attacking people. It's the energy that sustains long-term activism without depleting your soul.

This is why Tapping for anger and frustration is so powerful. When you tap through these emotions and begin to release their charge, when you interrupt those familiar patterns of frustration at the Choice Point, you open up new doors for what happens next.

And when you do that, when you create a new Rewired Response, here's what you can expect to experience:

- **Clarity and Strategy:** Instead of seeing everything through the lens of "this is wrong," you can assess situations objectively. You can distinguish between what's harmful and what's just different. You can think long term and find creative solutions.
- **Values-Based Response:** When you're not hijacked by reactivity, you can ask: "What action aligns with my values?" You can address problems without attacking people. You can stand up for what matters without burning bridges.

- **Sustainable Effectiveness:** Whether it's family dynamics or social justice, you can show up consistently without burning out. The world needs your sustained engagement, not your exhausted rage.

Consider what happened to Caroline. She wrote in to tell us about using Tapping in a situation that had made her unexpectedly angry—a situation in which she felt excluded and left out. She told us, "I was able to tap on the anger I was feeling, which I don't normally feel. I let go of the feeling of being excluded and had a vision of more expansive places I could be instead." Isn't that beautiful? When the anger cleared, vision and possibilities emerged where Caroline could step forward as her authentic self.

Or, take Grace. After tapping on her anger at a hurtful comment her boss made, she told us, "A day or two later, I feel sorry for her lack of heart and care. I wonder what life experiences have led her to be this way." She moved from fury to compassion without becoming a doormat.

This same pattern played out for Charissa, who shared: "After two or three months of Tapping often on finances and releasing negative emotions, I got really angry that my considerable skills were benefiting others more than they were benefiting me. . . . It was that anger that flipped the switch for me to move forward, and a month after that, I was self-employed, more than doubling my income without any negative side-effects."

For Caroline, Grace, and Charissa, the anger wasn't the enemy; it was valuable information. Once they could feel it without drowning in it, it became rocket fuel for change.

What is your anger or frustration trying to tell you? How would you show up differently if you could acknowledge it, then release it?

The Choice Point You Face Every Day

Every time you feel that familiar heat rising, when your co-worker e-mails in "sick" again, when you read another story that makes your blood boil, when someone says something that cuts deep, you're at a **Choice Point**.

You can choose the **Familiarity Trap**: Get frustrated, let it ruin your mood, carry that irritation into your next interaction, and reinforce the neural pathway that says, "The world is working against me."

Or you can choose to **Interrupt** the pattern. To pause. To breathe. To tap. To ask yourself: "What's actually happening here? What do I value? What action would align with who I want to be?"

Here's what becomes possible when you start interrupting your frustration patterns:

- **Morning Dishwasher Scenario, Rewired:** You open the dishwasher and see the plates facing the wrong way. You feel the familiar irritation starting to rise. You pause, start tapping, and think: "This is just how they load dishwashers. What matters more right now, being right or being connected?" You choose connection, mention it kindly later, and your morning stays peaceful.

- **Workplace Frustration, Rewired:** Your co-worker calls in "sick" again before a major deadline. Your blood starts to boil. But you tap and breathe, saying to yourself, "This pattern affects the team. I can either complain about it or address it professionally. What's the most effective response here?" You document the pattern, talk to your boss. Change begins.
- **News Story Reaction, Rewired:** You read something that makes your blood boil—another story of injustice or cruelty. You feel the rage building. You begin tapping and ask yourself, "How can I channel this energy into something constructive? What action aligns with my values?" You donate, call your representative, or volunteer. Anger becomes fuel for positive change.
- **Personal Slight, Rewired:** Someone says something that hurts your feelings. Your first instinct is to attack back or withdraw completely. As you start tapping, you say to yourself, "That hurt. What response honors my boundaries and values?" You have a direct conversation about impact, set a clear boundary, and maintain your integrity.
- **Traffic Moment, Rewired:** You're stuck behind someone going 10 mph under the speed limit. Your blood pressure starts rising. But you start tapping: "They're driving their comfort level. I can rage or use this time well." You call your mom, listen to a podcast, or practice gratitude.

The Life That Waits on the Other Side

What if you could go through your day without being hijacked by every small inefficiency or major injustice? What if other people's choices didn't automatically become your emotional emergency? What if you could care deeply about things without being consumed by rage about them?

Here's what people discover when they rewire their frustration patterns:

- Your relationships improve dramatically. Your family feels safer around you.
- Your energy returns for actually making positive changes.
- Your health improves. Lower stress hormones, better sleep, lower blood pressure.
- Your effectiveness increases. People listen more because you're not constantly outraged.
- Your perspective expands. The world becomes more nuanced—still imperfect, but not hopeless.

Chris discovered what 71 years of warehousing anger was costing her after she started Tapping. She found herself called to tap on anger, and remarkable changes started to occur in her life and in her body: "My BP is going down, and stress eating is decreasing."

Her body had been taking a toll, and as soon as the anger was let go, her body let go right along with it.

Annika discovered: "I have noticed such a lightness, and things that used to make me super angry are now only a ripple."

Luke transformed completely: "I used to get so angry with family members. Tapping has helped me to relax into life, to trust, to go with flow. I can now process my emotions and show up in life the way I want, with more energy and joy."

Sandra found unexpected forgiveness: "I felt a sense of softening and forgiveness towards everyone . . . and had more realizations that I can create strategies, plus that I can cope!"

The Invitation to Everyday Peace

The frustration you've been carrying isn't serving you or the world. It's not making you more effective or protecting you from disappointment. It's just making you more miserable.

You don't have to like inefficiency. You don't have to approve of unfairness. You don't have to stop caring about what matters.

But you can choose not to let other people's choices hijack your nervous system. You can choose to respond instead of react. You can choose to care deeply without carrying frustration everywhere you go.

Your co-worker will still have questionable work habits. Politicians will still disappoint you. People will still sometimes hurt your feelings. Injustice will still exist.

But you? You can move through it all with your inner calm intact and your effectiveness increased. You can be the person who doesn't get thrown off by life's imperfections. You can be the one who stays centered in the chaos while actually creating positive change.

That's not just possible—it's your power.

Ready to stop being at the mercy of every annoyance and injustice? Ready to transform your anger into effective action?

Let's tap.

RECLAIMING *Your* FREEDOMS

The pattern we explored in this chapter doesn't just cause discomfort; it actively steals some of your 7 Freedoms. By using Tapping to rewire this pattern, you're not just getting rid of a problem–you're reclaiming your birthright to a full, vibrant life.

Take a moment to reflect: Which of these freedoms would open up the most for you if this pattern no longer had a hold on you?

- The freedom to experience emotions without being overwhelmed.
- The freedom to respond with wisdom instead of reacting from old wounds.
- The freedom to feel calm in situations that used to throw you.
- The freedom to access energy you didn't know you had.
- The freedom to feel at home and peaceful in your body.
- The freedom to trust yourself to handle whatever comes your way.
- The freedom to show up as your real self, not who you've been conditioned to be.

What is the first thing you would do, create, or experience with this newfound freedom?

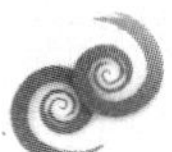

TAPPING SCRIPT: *Breaking Free from Frustration Patterns*

Let's take a moment to check in.

How are you feeling about life's daily annoyances? Is there something recently that's been getting under your skin? Give your current frustration level a number from 0 to 10, where 10 is "I'm feeling completely bothered" and 0 is "I feel patient and peaceful."

Take a gentle breath in . . . and out.

Start tapping on the side of your hand. Repeat either in your mind or out loud.

Side of the Hand: Even though I've noticed this pattern
of getting frustrated easily,
and sometimes things really get to me,
I acknowledge how I feel.

Even though certain things really bother me,
And I wish I knew how to handle them better,
I choose to be kind to myself right now.

Even though I wish things would go more smoothly,
I choose to slow down and breathe deeply now.

Eyebrow: These feelings of frustration
Side of the Eye: Things that get under my skin
Under the Eye: One thing after another
Under the Nose: Sometimes life feels unfair . . .
Under the Mouth: and I wish things were different
Collarbone: This tension builds up inside
Under the Arm: I sometimes try to ignore it
Top of the Head: But it still affects how I show up

Eyebrow: What if I could step back for a moment . . .
Side of the Eye: and safely reflect?
Under the Eye: What is really bothering me?
Under the Nose: Maybe it's the lack of control?
Under the Mouth: Wanting to make things different?

Collarbone: Feeling stuck or powerless?
Under the Arm: I notice what comes up for me
Top of the Head: I've been holding on to a lot

Eyebrow: It's okay to have these feelings
Side of the Eye: They're an invitation to check in . . .
Under the Eye: and tune in to what feels right for me
Under the Nose: I give myself space . . .
Under the Mouth: for clarity to arise
Collarbone: I act from a grounded place
Under the Arm: I'm open to new ideas and possibilities
Top of the Head: I can navigate what's ahead of me

Eyebrow: I don't need all the answers now
Side of the Eye: Clarity is on its way
Under the Eye: And for now, it's safe to rest
Under the Nose: Giving my mind and body a break
Under the Mouth: Releasing any excess tension . . .
Collarbone: and finding my center
Under the Arm: Feeling safe and grounded
Top of the Head: Feeling capable and ready

Gently stop tapping and let your hands rest. Take a deep breath in . . . and let it out slowly.

Check back in with yourself now. Where's your frustration level on that 0-to-10 scale? Notice how even a small shift gives you more space to respond thoughtfully.

You've just proven that frustration doesn't have to ruin your day. And now, new ideas and possibilities are on their way.

For a guided audio version of this Tapping meditation, visit www.thetappingsolution.com/rewired.

To Remember . . .

The Core Insight: *The peace you're seeking isn't found in controlling everything around you. It's found in changing your relationship with life's imperfections and injustices. You have the choice to stop being controlled by your reactivity and instead become someone who turns raw anger into focused, constructive action.*

The Practice: *Use the flash of anger as your signal to begin your practice. Instead of letting it spiral, immediately tap on the charge of the emotion. Every time you tap instead of fume, you're training your nervous system that you're safe and have agency even when life isn't perfect and the world isn't fair. This empowers you to respond with clarity and strength.*

CHAPTER 7

When You Feel Numb

Finding Your Way Back to Feeling

You know this feeling.

Or rather, you don't. And that's precisely the problem.

It's a Tuesday evening. Nothing terrible has happened today. Nothing wonderful either. You should be feeling . . . something. But instead, there's this vague emptiness. A peculiar hollowness that's somehow become more familiar than any specific emotion.

You go through the motions of daily life. You smile when appropriate. You respond when spoken to. You meet deadlines. You prepare meals. From the outside, you appear completely functional and normal.

But inside? There's a foggy window between you and the world. You can see life happening—people laughing, crying, celebrating, connecting—but you can't quite reach it clearly. You're watching a movie of your own life with the volume turned down and the colors desaturated.

This emotional numbness is a specific type of Reactive Loop, one I call the "shutdown loop." It's your nervous system's most extreme protective measure, essentially pulling the emergency brake on all feeling to prevent overwhelm.

Someone asks, "How are you?" and you answer "Fine" automatically, because that seems like the easiest and most truthful answer. It's all just a little numb.

And maybe *numb* isn't your word. But maybe you recognize a "flattening" of your emotions, or areas of your life where you just can't seem to access as much joy or excitement or energy as you once had.

Maybe you've gotten so good at the performance that sometimes you fool even yourself. For a moment, you almost believe your own "I'm fine." Until you're alone again and the emptiness returns, reliable as gravity.

"I'M FINE" *and* OTHER COMMON PHRASES

Pause for a moment. Which of these phrases have become part of your vocabulary?

- "I'm fine."
- "I don't care."
- "Whatever."
- "It is what it is."
- "I'm just tired."
- "All good."

How often do you hear yourself saying these? Daily? Multiple times a day?

Notice what happens in your body when you say them. The slight shrug. The forced smile. The way your voice goes flat. The exhausted sigh that follows.

When did these become your go-to responses?

If you recognize yourself here, you're not alone. In fact, you're part of something much bigger.

The Epidemic No One Talks About

Here's a statistic that should make you sit up straighter: **21 million adults in the United States had at least one major depressive episode in a single year.** That's nearly 1 in 10 people walking around feeling disconnected from their own lives.

But here's what those numbers don't capture: the millions more who don't meet clinical criteria for "major depression" but wake up each day feeling like they're watching their lives through glass. People who function fine on the outside—show up to work, pay their bills, maintain relationships—while inside, they feel like emotional zombies.

This emotional numbness, this protective Reactive Loop of disconnection, has become so common, we've forgotten it's not normal. It's part of that Great Forgetting I talk about; we don't even remember what it's like to *not* feel this way.

This numbness loop has become so normalized that we've forgotten what it's like to have full access to our emotional spectrum. We've forgotten that feeling, even difficult feelings, is what makes us human.

Adrienne knew this experience intimately. "I've been feeling pretty flat lately," she wrote to us, "not interested in anything, hearing myself thinking 'I just don't care' numerous times a day every day."

I just don't care.

Four words that capture the essence of emotional numbness perfectly. Not "I'm devastated" or "I'm terrified" or "I'm furious." Just . . . nothing. The emotional equivalent of a shrug.

Those four words—"I just don't care"—aren't her truth. They're her shutdown loop running on autopilot, a Reactive Loop where the nervous system has decided that feeling nothing is safer than feeling anything.

The Brilliant Opossum

Let's talk about one of nature's most brilliant and misunderstood actors: the humble opossum. When an opossum is cornered by a threat it can't fight or outrun, it doesn't just pretend to be dead. It performs an involuntary, Oscar-worthy biological masterpiece. Its body goes limp, its heart rate plummets, and it even secretes a fluid that mimics the scent of death. It has become so overwhelmed that its nervous system makes a radical executive decision: Shut everything down. Feel nothing. Survive.

At some point in your own life, perhaps life began to feel like too much. The stress, the grief, the disappointment, the constant onslaught of to-dos. . . . It all felt like a predator you couldn't escape.

So your nervous system, in its infinite wisdom, did the only thing it could to protect you: It froze. It played dead. Your heart rate drops, your breathing slows, and most importantly, your emotional processing centers go offline. The problem is, unlike the opossum who shakes it off and scurries away once the coast is clear, you've stayed frozen long after the danger has passed.

You're playing dead in a life that's patiently waiting for you to live it.

The Worst Advice in the World

Let me tell you about the worst advice emotionally numb people receive:

"Just choose to be happy!" "Focus on gratitude!" "Fake it till you make it!" "You need to snap out of it!"

Ah yes, because emotional numbness is clearly just a case of forgetting to flip your happiness switch.

If you could "just choose" to feel, you would have done it already. Trust me, nobody volunteers for the cardboard cutout life.

Here's what people don't understand: Numbness isn't a choice or a character flaw. It's not laziness or ingratitude. It's your nervous system's version of a circuit breaker—it flips off to prevent the whole house from burning down.

So here's what I need you to know right now: This isn't permanent. This isn't "just who you are." It's a Familiarity Trap, sure. But it's also a nervous system pattern that can be changed. Not through willpower or positive thinking, but through a simple process that speaks directly to the part of your brain keeping you frozen. You have more agency here than you realize.

The Prison of "Safety"

Let's be honest. If you're feeling numb, part of you is terrified of what would happen if true feelings, true emotions returned. Numbness feels like a necessary shield, a form of safety from a world that proved to be too painful. And you're not wrong—it *is* a protective mechanism. It's a Familiarity Trap at its finest.

But why should you care about dismantling a wall that's keeping you safe?

Because that wall doesn't just block out pain. It blocks out *everything*. The price of admission to the prison of numbness is your entire life force.

- **It erases your inner compass.** How can you know what you want in life—in your career, your relationships, your day-to-day—if you can't *feel* it? Joy, excitement, and desire are your guidance system. Without them, you're just drifting.
- **It makes true connection impossible.** You can go through the motions of love and friendship, but without access to your own feelings, you can't truly connect with someone else's. You're an actor playing the part of a partner, a parent, or a friend.

- **It silences your intuition.** That gut feeling, that inner knowing—it's an emotional and somatic experience. When you're numb, you're cut off from one of the most powerful sources of wisdom you possess.

So, yes, letting feeling back in is a risk. But the "safety" of numbness has a 100 percent certainty: a life half-lived.

Numbness isn't protecting you from life—it's preventing you from living.

This chapter is your guide to turning the lights back on, not with a blinding flood, but one dimmer switch at a time, until you can navigate your life not by thought alone, but with the full, colorful, and wise spectrum of human emotion.

When 20 Years of Tears Finally Fall

Marta knew this prison intimately. For years, she'd been her husband's sole caregiver through his terminal illness. When the doctors gave the news that he had only one year left, she left her job to be by his side for what she thought would be their final months together. That year stretched into seven.

"I was tired of having to do so much," she told us later, "but I was full of love for my husband." The guilt of feeling exhausted, the shame of wanting it to be over, the anger at their situation . . . they all felt like too much. Too complicated, too much to deal with when she already had so much on her plate.

So she did what felt safest: She pushed it all down.

When COVID hit and she found herself sick, grieving, and more burned out than ever, a friend sent her a link to The Tapping Solution. And like many of us do when we have hit rock bottom and will try anything to find even a bit of relief, she decided to give Tapping a chance.

And it was like a floodgate opened. Tapping helped her finally give herself permission to feel it all. "It's okay that I feel all the feelings that I have in this moment. I'm not perfect, and it's okay to feel angry, to feel tired, to feel that I can't do any more."

All the things she'd been burying. All the feelings she'd been putting off—from her husband's illness and even before that—she finally, in the safe container of her Tapping practice, was able to let it all out.

"After tapping, I cried more tears at once than I had in twenty years," Marta told us.

The emotions she'd been protecting herself from? They weren't the enemy. They were just human responses to an impossibly difficult situation. They didn't make her a bad wife or a selfish person. They made her real.

The prison of numbness had felt like safety, but it was actually keeping her from the one thing that could truly free her: feeling her truth, letting it move through her, and discovering she could survive it—more than survive it, she could finally live again.

In her exact words: "It was like I was full of feelings, and after that I was free."

Full of feelings. Then free.

That's the journey from numbness to aliveness: not emptying yourself of emotion, but finally, safely, letting it flow through you.

The more Marta tapped, the more shifts she experienced. In her body, in her sense of self-worth, in her ability to access a sense of peace. . . .

"I deserve to be in this world," she now says. "Tapping changed my life."

Remember: Rewire

Remember: *How you've always felt isn't how you have to keep feeling. Who you've been isn't who you have to stay.*

Every trigger is a ***Choice Point****.*

Every pattern is just a ***Familiarity Trap****.*

And every tap is you choosing to ***Rewire*** *instead of repeat.*

Your Nervous System's Emergency Protocol

Here's what's actually happening in your brain and body when you feel numb:

Your nervous system has essentially hit the emergency brake. When life becomes too much to process—whether through trauma, chronic stress, or emotional overload—your system makes an executive decision: "We're shutting down nonessential functions to preserve energy for survival."

When you're stuck in emotional numbness, here's the biological reality:

- Your dorsal vagal system (the "shutdown" branch) is dominant
- Your limbic system's emotional processing becomes dysregulated, leading to blunted or numbed responses
- Your prefrontal cortex struggles to integrate experiences
- Neurotransmitters like dopamine and serotonin are dysregulated

- Your window of tolerance (ability to handle emotions) has narrowed to almost nothing

And what does that translate to? You may feel heavy, numb, foggy, and disconnected, as though your body is weighed down and your thoughts are far away. Emotionally, it can feel like being detached from life, unable to access joy, motivation, or even fear in a normal way, just a sense of flatness or being "offline."

For Marta, those 20 years of accumulated stress had pushed her system into permanent emergency mode.

Feeling becomes "nonessential." Not just the "hard" feelings, but the good ones too. Pleasure also becomes "nonessential." Joy, curiosity, excitement, connection—all filed under "luxury items we can't afford right now."

It's like your phone going into battery-saver mode. The screen dims, the background apps close, the notifications stop—everything designed to keep the device running but with minimal functionality.

The problem? Unlike your phone, you don't get a clear notification that you're in "survival mode" with an option to switch back. You just find yourself going through life at half-brightness, wondering where all the colors went.

The Three Settings Your Nervous System Operates On

Time for a quick science lesson (don't worry, there won't be a test).

Your nervous system has three main settings:

1. **"Life is good" mode (ventral vagal):** You're connected, present, able to feel the full spectrum of emotions. This is you at your best—laughing with friends, crying at movies, feeling genuinely excited about pizza night.
2. **"Danger! Danger!" mode (sympathetic):** Fight or flight. Heart racing, muscles tensed, ready for action. This is you when someone cuts you off in traffic or when you realize you forgot about that big presentation.
3. **"Play dead" mode (dorsal vagal):** Total shutdown. Disconnection. Numbness. This is your nervous system's last resort when it decides the situation is hopeless.

Here's the kicker: In nature, animals shake off the "play dead" response within minutes. Like opossums, who play dead to avoid a predator. Once safe, they shudder and reset, discharging the freeze response, then scurry away like nothing happened.

Humans? We can stay frozen for years.

Why? Because we have this pesky thing called a prefrontal cortex that creates stories about our experiences. Instead of shaking it off like the gazelle, we think thoughts like:

"I should be over this by now." "What's wrong with me?" "I'm broken." "This is just who I am now."

And those thoughts keep us stuck in freeze mode, like a computer trapped in an endless reboot cycle.

This is where numbness becomes a **Reactive Loop**—your nervous system's automated response to emotional overload. Every morning you wake up and unconsciously choose the familiar numbness over the unknown territory of feeling.

It's the Familiarity Trap at its most insidious: Your system would rather stay in the prison it knows than risk the freedom it doesn't.

But you're not actually trapped. You're just running an outdated program. And with Tapping, you can Recognize when the numbness kicks in, Interrupt the shutdown sequence, and Rewire your response to life's emotional content.

Research Spotlight

When researchers study Tapping for depression, they consistently find something remarkable: effect sizes that dwarf what we see with traditional treatments.

A recent meta-analysis of 18 studies found that Tapping produced an effect size of 1.27 for depression. To put that in perspective, antidepressant medications typically show effect sizes of 0.3 to 0.5, and psychotherapy usually ranges from 0.6 to 0.8.[9]

An effect size of 1.27 means that many people moved from clinical depression to normal functioning.

The Science That Changes Everything: The Paradox of Feeling to Heal

If you've been struggling with numbness, you've probably tried things. Maybe therapy, meditation, exercise, gratitude journaling, or even medication. Some might have helped a little, giving you tools for managing daily life or helping you understand your patterns better.

But if you're reading this chapter, I'm guessing you're still searching for that thing that actually brings you back to life.

Here's something that might sound counterintuitive: **To restore your ability to feel good, you first have to be willing to feel bad.**

Numbness isn't the absence of emotion, it's the *suppression* of emotion.

Somewhere underneath that protective shutdown, all your feelings are still there, waiting. The sadness, yes, but also the anger, the fear, the disappointment that you couldn't process when it was happening.

But also the joy, the love, the excitement, the hope that got buried along with everything else.

Tapping works for numbness because it provides a safe way to begin feeling again. The physical act of Tapping signals safety to your nervous system while you gently bring your attention to what's there underneath the protective shutdown.

It's like slowly turning up the lights in a room that's been dark for a long time. You don't flip them on all at once—that would be overwhelming. You gradually adjust the dimmer until you can see clearly again.

It's like every morning when I wake up my three-year-old son, Ellis. If I just turn on the lights full blast, he yells, "Too bright!" Instead, I open the door wide, pull back the shades partway to let some natural light in, and turn on a small lamp—so he can adjust to a new day.

THE LAW OF EMERGENCE

When we start to come back to life from numbness, it doesn't always feel good at first. This is governed by a crucial concept I call the **Law of Emergence**.

THE RULE:
When suppressed emotions emerge, it is not a setback; it is progress.

Think about what happens when a frozen limb begins to thaw: It aches and burns. That pain isn't a sign of new damage; it's the feeling of life returning to the nerves. The same is true for your emotional system.

After years of protective numbness, the return of feeling, even if it's sadness or anger, is the return of your life force. It's not a sign you're getting worse; it's the first, brave sign that you're starting to heal.

You Don't Have to Feel It All at Once

If you've been numb for weeks, months, or years, the thought of feeling again might be terrifying. What if the pain is unbearable? What if you can't handle what's underneath the numbness?

Here's your permission slip: You don't have to feel everything at once. Tapping allows you to titrate the process—to feel just a little bit at a time, in a safe and controlled way.

You're not jumping into the deep end of emotion. You're wading in gradually, with support, with tools, with the ability to slow down or stop whenever you need to.

Think of it like physical therapy after an injury. You don't try to run a marathon on day one. You start with gentle movements, building strength and flexibility gradually until you can handle more.

Your emotional system works the same way. It needs gentle, consistent practice to remember how to feel again.

Remember Adrienne, from earlier? The one who kept feeling "flat" and heard herself thinking "I just don't care" numerous times per day?

Well, here's what happened for her after Tapping.

She wrote to us: "**I feel alive again!** It's not like some miraculous recovery or anything, but I have to say I'm absolutely loving feeling SOMETHING right now."

Read that line again: "I'm absolutely loving feeling SOMETHING right now."

That's what happens when the emotional volume starts coming back up. Not a dramatic, overwhelming, unbearable tidal wave, but an encouraging, empowering, first flicker of life returning to a system that had previously gone quiet.

Your Road Map Back to Feeling

Unlike the movies where someone has a breakthrough and suddenly feels everything in one cathartic moment, most of the time healing follows a more gentle arc.

Based on thousands of reports from people who've used Tapping to emerge from numbness, here's what you might experience:

The First Flickers (Days 1–14)

- Moments where you notice you're feeling something, even if it's sadness or irritation

- Brief periods where colors seem a little brighter
- Catching yourself actually laughing at something (and being surprised by it)
- Feeling more present in conversations, even if just for minutes at a time

The Volume Increases (Weeks 3–4)

- Emotions start feeling less muffled
- You might cry, possibly for the first time in months or years
- Anger might surface (this is actually good news, because anger is life-force energy)
- Interest in things might start to return, even faintly

The Range Expands (Month 2–3)

- Bad days feel genuinely sad rather than empty
- Good moments start to feel genuinely good
- You begin to care about outcomes again
- Decision making becomes easier because you can feel your preferences

The Life Returns (Month 3+)

- Emotional responses feel proportionate to situations
- You rediscover what you actually enjoy
- Relationships feel more connecting because you're more present
- Purpose and meaning start to emerge naturally

You won't suddenly feel everything at once (that would be overwhelming and counterproductive). Instead, you'll experience what I call "the gradual dawn"—colors slowly returning to a black-and-white world. Some days you'll feel more, some days less.

Ephiny experienced this progression: "Honestly, the first time I started tapping with this app made me realize that I benefit from it every time. I struggle with anxiety, depression, getting up in the mornings and having energy. This app has never let me down!"

Notice how her challenges didn't disappear, but her relationship to them transformed. She went from struggling against depression to having a tool that never lets her down. From being at the mercy of her emotional state to having reliable access to feeling better.

The Invisible Recovery

Genine understood the prison of numbness well. She was dealing with major depression and anxiety, compounded by the death of her father. But here's what makes her story remarkable: "Even the mention of the word *tapping* and I feel relaxed and in control."

Notice that phrase: "I feel relaxed and in control." For someone who had been struggling with major depression, just the word *tapping* became associated with the possibility of feeling something other than numb or overwhelmed.

"I have been tapping for a while now, and whilst I still have bad days, overall, I am in a better place mentally than I have been in a long time."

This is what recovery from numbness actually looks like. Not perfect days. Not constant happiness. But the return of emotional range; good days and bad days instead of just flat days.

That's your nervous system learning a new association. Instead of feeling powerless against emotional numbness, you start to have a tool that consistently brings you back to yourself.

The Return of Your Essential Self

Numbness isn't protecting you, it's stealing your life. You're missing your actual existence. Your kids are growing up, seasons are changing, life is happening—and you're watching it all through bulletproof glass.

What waits for you on the other side of numbness isn't just the ability to feel emotions again. It's the return of your essential self, the person you were before life taught you that feeling wasn't safe.

That person who had opinions about things. Who got excited about possibilities. Who felt moved by music, sunsets, or a friend's good news. Who cared about outcomes because they could feel the difference between good and bad, meaningful and empty, connected and alone.

That person isn't gone. They're just behind the protective wall your nervous system built. And every time you tap, you're gently letting them know it's safe to come out again.

RECLAIMING *Your* FREEDOMS

The pattern we explored in this chapter doesn't just cause discomfort; it actively steals some of your 7 Freedoms. By using Tapping to rewire this pattern, you're not just getting rid of a problem, you're reclaiming your birthright to a full, vibrant life.

Take a moment to reflect: Which of these freedoms would open up the most for you if this pattern no longer had a hold on you?

- The freedom to experience emotions without being overwhelmed.
- The freedom to respond with wisdom instead of reacting from old wounds.
- The freedom to feel calm in situations that used to throw you.
- The freedom to access energy you didn't know you had.
- The freedom to feel at home and peaceful in your body.
- The freedom to trust yourself to handle whatever comes your way.
- The freedom to show up as your real self, not who you've been conditioned to be.

What is the first thing you would do, create, or experience with this newfound freedom?

Your Invitation Back to Life

So here you are, sitting with that glass wall between you and the world, reading about people who found their way back to feeling. Maybe part of you is thinking, "That sounds nice, but I've been this way for so long. What if I'm just not capable of feeling deeply anymore?"

I understand that fear. When you've been numb for a long time, it starts to feel like your permanent address rather than a temporary shelter.

But here's what I know after working with thousands of people: Your capacity to feel isn't broken. It's just protected. And protection can be gently, gradually lifted when it's no longer needed.

The research is clear: Tapping can help lift depression with effect sizes larger than traditional antidepressants. The stories are consistent: People rediscover their capacity for joy, connection, and purpose. The tool is simple enough that you can start right now.

You don't have to stay behind that glass wall. You don't have to settle for watching your life happen from the outside. You don't have to accept that "this is just how you are."

Your feelings are waiting for you. Not the overwhelming, scary feelings you might be imagining, but the full spectrum of human experience, including joy, curiosity, love, and hope.

Your life is waiting for you. Your essential self, the one who knows how to be fully present, fully alive, is waiting for you.

Ready to turn up the volume on life again?

Let's tap.

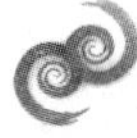

TAPPING SCRIPT: *Reconnecting to Yourself*

Let's check in with how you're feeling emotionally right now.

On a scale of 0 to 10, where 10 is feeling completely numb or disconnected and 0 is feeling clear and connected, where are you?

Take a gentle breath in . . . and out.

Start tapping on the side of your hand. Repeat either in your mind or out loud.

Side of the Hand: Even though I haven't been feeling much lately,
I acknowledge where I am right now.

Even though life feels a bit muted or distant,
like I'm going through the motions,
I'm open to gently reconnecting with myself.

Even though part of me might be scared to feel fully again,
because it might be overwhelming,
I choose to be patient and gentle with myself.

When You Feel Numb

Eyebrow: This disconnected feeling
Side of the Eye: Like life is happening at a distance
Under the Eye: Going through the motions
Under the Nose: Not feeling as much joy as I used to
Under the Mouth: Sometimes feeling nothing at all
Collarbone: This protective numbness
Under the Arm: My heart feels a bit closed
Top of the Head: Like I've been living behind glass

Eyebrow: I acknowledge this is just my brain . . .
Side of the Eye: trying to protect me
Under the Eye: But I now know I am safe
Under the Nose: It is safe to feel again
Under the Mouth: I can explore all my feelings . . .
Collarbone: with curiosity and compassion
Under the Arm: I reassure the parts of me that are scared . . .
Top of the Head: and appreciate the parts that are hopeful

Eyebrow: I don't have to control every feeling
Side of the Eye: I'm open to seeing what comes up . . .
Under the Eye: without judgment
Under the Nose: There's room for all my feelings
Under the Mouth: I see the good intentions behind my feelings . . .
Collarbone: and find more ease within them
Under the Arm: Allowing these feelings to move through me
Top of Head: I'm gently opening up
Eyebrow: I'm open to new possibilities

Side of the Eye: I notice little sparks of interest
Under the Eye: A flicker of joy here
Under the Nose: A moment of connection there
Under the Mouth: I'm coming back to life
Collarbone: My inner world is waking up
Under the Arm: Coming back to myself
Top of the Head: It is safe to feel again

Gently stop tapping and let your hands rest. Take a deep breath in . . . and let it out slowly.

Check in with yourself now. Where are you on that 0-to-10 scale? Even a small shift toward feeling more alive and in touch with your emotions is your nervous system remembering it's safe to feel.

You're not broken. Your ability to feel joy, excitement, and connection is still there, just waiting for the right moment to return. And that moment might be now.

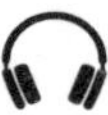

For a guided audio version of this Tapping meditation, visit www.thetappingsolution.com/rewired.

To Remember . . .

The Core Insight: *Numbness is not an empty void; it is a protective fortress your nervous system built to survive an overwhelming experience. The hopeful truth is that your capacity for joy and connection isn't gone; it is simply dormant, waiting inside for a clear signal that it is finally safe to emerge.*

The Practice: *Your practice is to become your own safe harbor. Gently tap not to force a feeling, but to prove your own trustworthiness to your nervous system. By tapping with phrases like, "I am safe in this moment," you are actively demonstrating that you can and will protect yourself, giving the frozen parts of you the confidence they need to thaw at their own pace.*

CHAPTER 8

When Fear Stops You Cold

Unlocking Courage in the Body

Your palms start to sweat. Your heart pounds against your ribs. Your breath catches in your throat. Every muscle in your body tenses, ready to run.

All because of . . . what, exactly?

Maybe it's the thought of getting on a plane. Perhaps it's a spider in the corner of your bedroom. It could be the elevator doors closing, the mere suggestion of speaking in front of a group, or walking through the doors of the dentist's office.

You know it's ridiculous.

Your rational mind is screaming: "This is insane! It's an elevator! Flying is statistically safer than driving! It's just a routine visit to get my teeth cleaned!"

But your body doesn't care about statistics. When something scary happens, your amygdala (the brain's fear center) gets the signal in just a few milliseconds—long before your "thinking brain" (the prefrontal cortex) has a chance to weigh in. By the time logic shows up a quarter of a second later, your nervous system has already hit the panic button, flooding you with adrenaline and screaming one message: DANGER!

This fear response, this particular type of Reactive Loop, is your amygdala hijacking your entire system based on outdated threat assessment. It's running a program written for actual survival threats but applying it to modern situations that are, indeed, safe.

You feel embarrassed. Frustrated. Maybe even angry at yourself. Because you *know* this doesn't make sense. You *know* you're being "irrational." But knowing doesn't help. Logic doesn't help. Understanding the facts doesn't help.

If anything, being aware of how "silly" your fear is makes it worse. Now you're not just afraid—you're ashamed of being afraid.

Here's what I want you to understand: That fear that's been running your life? That's not your permanent identity. That's just a fear-based Reactive Loop—old programming that can be updated. And I'm about to show you exactly how.

THE LAW OF SOMATIC PRIORITY (THE BODY VETOES THE BRAIN)

If fear has shown up in your life, and it doesn't even feel logical, know this: You're simply experiencing a nonnegotiable truth of how you are wired. This is one of the most important laws of your nervous system: the **Law of Somatic Priority**.

THE RULE:
When your logical mind and your survival brain (nervous system) disagree, the survival brain always wins.

You cannot *think* your way out of a *feeling* problem. Your conscious mind can have all the statistics about flight safety, but if your body *feels* unsafe, your body will win that argument 100 percent of the time. It has veto power. This is why positive thinking and logical reassurances fail against deep fear. To change the fear, you must speak the language of the body. Tapping is that language.

The Loyal Soldier Still on Patrol

Decades after World War II ended in 1945, a handful of Japanese soldiers, hidden deep in the jungles of remote Pacific islands, continued to fight. They were completely cut off from the chain of command, so they never received the message that the war was over. With unwavering loyalty, they kept running patrols, maintaining their weapons, and defending their posts from perceived enemies. They were perfect soldiers, running on the last, most urgent command they had received: "We are at war."

It wasn't until as late as the 1970s that the last of these "holdouts" were found and gently convinced by former commanders and family members that it was finally safe to come home.

Your nervous system, in its own profound loyalty, can sometimes inadvertently become a "holdout." After a difficult or traumatic event–a painful breakup, a deep betrayal, a scary accident–it receives the urgent command: "We are under attack! Never let this happen again!"

Long after the conflict is over, a part of you remains in the jungle of your past, on high alert. You can't heal by shouting at this loyal soldier to give up. You have to send a trusted envoy to meet them right where they are and respectfully show them that the danger has passed.

The Prison Built from One Moment

Octavia had been living according to a program written in terror for years.

It started when her six-year-old son was bitten by a dog during a family camping trip. One moment of terror—a dog jumping up, her child's scream, blood on his face—and her nervous system installed a new operating system.

The irony? Her son bounced back fine. Kids are resilient like that. He showed no lasting fear of dogs whatsoever. His system processed the experience and moved on.

But Octavia's nervous system had written a different program. As she described it: "I would become terrified if I even saw a dog in the distance and could not move or breathe."

Think about what that would be like for a moment. A dog in the *distance*. Not approaching. Not barking. Not showing any signs of aggression. Just . . . existing in her field of vision, and her entire system would lock up.

Her world had shrunk accordingly. No visiting friends with dogs. No walking in parks. No outdoor events where dogs might appear. This is what happens when old programming runs your life: It doesn't just limit one area, it redesigns everything.

Octavia's story perfectly illustrates how a single moment can install a fear-based Reactive Loop that runs for years. Here's what happened neurologically: In that moment of terror, her amygdala created what researchers call a "flashbulb memory"—an intensely encoded memory tagged as critical for survival. Every time she saw a dog after that, her nervous system ran the same program: Dog detected → Amygdala fires → Full fear response initiated → Avoid at all costs.

And over time, she got stuck in that **Familiarity Trap**. Avoiding dogs became Octavia's normal. Planning routes to avoid parks, declining invitations, having to cross to the other side of the street on every walk—it all became familiar, therefore "safe." Her nervous system preferred the prison of limitation to the uncertainty of change. But limitation isn't safety, it's just familiar suffering.

But here's what Octavia later discovered (we'll return to the rest of her story later) that should give you incredible hope: **Programs can be rewritten. Reactive Loops can be interrupted. Old wiring can be updated.**

And sometimes it happens faster than you ever imagined possible.

When 25 Years of Terror Meets 15 Minutes of Tapping

Christian's story shows just how deeply these old programs can run—and how dramatically they can change.

For 25 years after a car accident in Botswana, Christian couldn't be a passenger in a car traveling over 50 miles per hour without experiencing pure terror. Racing heart. Dizziness. The absolute certainty of impending death.

He could drive just fine. That felt different because he had control. But as a passenger? His nervous system would flood with panic every single time.

It was always there. Not just in Botswana, but back home in Germany. Anywhere he went. That background anxiety that started the minute he was sitting in the passenger seat, and that would spike into panic around curves or at certain speeds. Christian just accepted this as how things were. Driving was a terrifying experience, and that's just how it would always be.

But what if 25 years of automatic terror could be updated in minutes?

When Christian finally worked with a therapist who used Tapping, something remarkable happened. The session took him directly back to the source, that moment in the Kalahari when the car began to swerve.

"After just 15 minutes of tapping and reactivating the feeling of the accident, which I experienced as if in slow motion, I was able to separate the emerging fear from the memory," he said. "So that I could only recall the memory, but no longer the feeling of swerving, of overturning, of the fear of the accident."

For 25 years, every time Christian remembered that accident, his body reacted as if it were happening again. The memory and the fear were fused together, inseparable.

And then, the Tapping. Tapping allowed him to keep the memory but release the fear—to finally file that experience in the past where it belonged.

"Just 15 minutes of tapping freed me from that. Now I can sit in the car as a passenger again and am (almost) never afraid anymore."

Twenty-five years of terror. Fifteen minutes of rewiring. A whole new life of freedom waiting to be explored.

You don't have to be stuck in the patterns that have always stuck you.

WHAT ARE YOU AFRAID OF?

What fear has become so baked into your identity that you've stopped questioning it and just accepted, "this is who I am"?

Common fears and phobias:

- ❑ Fear of driving
- ❑ Fear of the doctor
- ❑ Fear of the dentist
- ❑ Fear of spiders
- ❑ Fear of needles
- ❑ Fear of heights
- ❑ Fear of small spaces
- ❑ Fear of public speaking
- ❑ Fear of water
- ❑ Fear of animals

The Original Phobia Cure

The story of Tapping begins with psychologist Dr. Roger Callahan and his patient Mary in the 1980s. We met Mary back in Chapter 3. As a reminder, Mary had such severe water phobia that she couldn't bathe her children or even handle a wet washcloth without panic. She had nightmares about water and couldn't go near swimming pools.

After 18 months of conventional therapy with little progress, Dr. Callahan tried something unconventional. Knowing that Mary felt her fear in her stomach, and having recently studied meridian points from traditional Chinese medicine, he asked her to tap under her eye–a point associated with the stomach meridian.

What happened next changed the course of psychology: Mary's lifelong phobia vanished. Not gradually. Instantly. She ran to his swimming pool and began splashing water on her face, laughing at the absurdity of her sudden freedom.

This "one-minute cure" seemed impossible, yet it was real and lasting. Mary's phobia never returned. Dr. Callahan went on to develop Thought Field Therapy, which eventually evolved into EFT (Emotional Freedom Techniques), the system used by millions today.

The skeptics were numerous–how could tapping on your face eliminate a phobia that years of therapy couldn't touch? But as research has accumulated and our understanding of memory reconsolidation has grown, Mary's miracle cure looks less like magic and more like neuroscience in action.

The Science of Getting Unstuck

Here's what's happening when you feel trapped by fear: Your brain has carved a superhighway between "trigger" and "terror," a classic Reactive Loop that fires automatically. Every time you encounter your fear object, traffic flows down this well-worn path automatically.

Dog appears → Path to Panic
Plane ticket bought → Time for Terror
Elevator doors close → Engage Escape Plan

You've been traveling these same neural highways for so long, you assume they're permanent. But they're not. They're just the most familiar route that you've gotten used to traveling over time.

Tapping builds new roads.

When you tap while thinking about your fear, something remarkable happens: You're simultaneously accessing the old program (thinking about dogs/planes/elevators) while introducing completely new information to your system (the calming signals from acupoint stimulation).

Your nervous system gets confused in the best possible way. It's like your brain saying: *"Wait, we're thinking about the scary thing but feeling calm? This doesn't match our programming. Let me update this file."*

And that's exactly what happens. The old program gets opened for editing, updated with new information, and saved as a new version.

The Memory Editing Revolution

Here's where the science gets really fascinating. In the early 2000s, neuroscientist Karim Nader made a discovery that revolutionized our understanding of memory. He found that when you recall a memory, it becomes temporarily unstable—essentially "unlocked" for editing.

Scientists call this "memory reconsolidation." Think of it like opening a document on your computer. While it's open, you can edit it. When you save and close it, the edited version becomes the new file.

Dr. Daniela Schiller at Mount Sinai puts it like this: "When you remember something, it can go back to an unstable state in the brain, and if it's not restored just as it was stored in the beginning, then it might be lost or modified."[10]

This is exactly what happened to Christian. When he recalled the car accident while tapping, that fear memory became temporarily editable. The Tapping provided new information—safety, calm, present-moment awareness—that got integrated with the old memory. When his brain "saved" the memory again, it was a new version: memory of an accident without all the fear and terror.

This explains why the results with Tapping can be so rapid and permanent. You're not just managing symptoms or building coping skills. You're rewriting the source code.

And that is exactly how we move from Reactive Loops to Rewired Responses. The old neural pathway (Dog = Extreme Danger) gets overwritten with new information (Dog = Safe/Neutral). Your Choice Point, that moment when you see a dog, transforms from automatic panic to conscious choice.

The Airport Rewiring (Yes, That Story Again)

Remember the woman from the Introduction? The one whose family was crying at the airport gate because her fear wouldn't let her board the plane to London. The one who, thanks to a kind stranger tapping with her, was able to release her fear and get on the plane?

Well, my brother, Alex, has his own airplane story that shows us that even at 30,000 feet with nowhere to run, you can still move through fear and find peace.

Alex was on a flight to Dallas for a speaking event with his wife, Karen. Everything seemed normal until a man rushed to the front of the plane, clearly in distress.

So much distress, in fact, that the flight attendants were talking with the captain about turning the plane around. This wasn't just mild nervousness; this was full-blown panic that could ground an entire flight.

Alex, watching this whole scene unfold, knew he had an opportunity to help.

He approached the flight attendant and explained that he worked with people experiencing anxiety. Could he help?

The attendant's relief was visible. "Please, try."

Alex went to the back of the plane and sat with the man in the very last row. For the next 20 minutes, Alex walked him through a Tapping session. Just two guys in the back of a plane, one teaching the other how to interrupt a panic pattern that had completely hijacked his nervous system.

"The shift was incredible after we did the Tapping. He was able to completely calm down," Alex said. "I stayed with him back there for the rest of the flight."

When the plane landed, paramedics checked the man out as a precaution. But he was fine. More than fine, in fact. He and Alex even took a picture, smiling together. An impromptu teacher-student pair who'd found each other at 30,000 feet.

Here's what strikes me about these stories. The woman at the gate in the Introduction received help from a stranger who knew Tapping. This man on Alex's flight received help from my brother. How many other mid-air interventions are happening as this movement spreads?

How many people are discovering that their worst fears can be interrupted and rewired, even in the very moment they're experiencing them?

Tapping for Fear of Flying: Breaking It Down

Here's what happened for the woman in the airport and the man on the plane that should change how you think about what's possible:

- **Old Reactive Loop Running:** Plane = Danger
- **Choice Point Hit:** Stranger offers Tapping. Completely unexpected input to the system.
- **Pattern Interrupt Chosen:** Despite the panic, the embarrassment, the newness of a technique, they tap through their fear and send calming signals to the nervous system.
- **System Update Complete. Fear, Rewired:** Now, Plane = Safe. Plane = A Form of Transportation. "I can get on that plane." or "I can make it through this flight." Family stays together. Man gets to his destination.

Ten to 20 minutes. One pattern interrupt. What had been a complete limitation, now rewired.

These people proved in just a few minutes what this entire book promises: **You don't have to be who you've always been.**

The Two-Session Revolution

Remember Octavia, the woman from earlier, whose child had been attacked by a dog? Well, she had been tapping on other issues for weeks when she decided it was time to challenge her fear of dogs programming. She understood how Tapping worked. She'd experienced the rewiring process on other issues in her life.

"In two self-administered Tapping sessions, my fear of dogs gradually released."

Two sessions were all it took. Done all on her own, with no specific training or special equipment. Just her, recognizing her fear Reactive Loop, choosing to interrupt it with Tapping, and rewiring her response to dogs.

And with that, years of limitation were reprogrammed.

But here's the beautiful part. Octavia went on to tell us, "I tested myself soon afterwards when a neighbor came toward me with her dog, and I did not freeze and panic as I normally did. A week later I let myself pet him and felt as if I had my life back again."

This is exactly why we do what we do, and why we are writing this book. *Octavia felt like she got her life back again.*

And isn't that what we all want? Don't we all just want to feel free to live our lives and enjoy them to the fullest?

Today, Octavia's son is 39 and married to a dog trainer. They have three dogs who are the first to greet Octavia when she goes to babysit her grandchildren.

From **Dogs = Extreme Danger** to **Dogs = Welcome Committee for Grandma.**

This is what becomes possible when you stop accepting old programming as permanent and start believing in the power of rewiring.

RECLAIMING *Your* FREEDOMS

The pattern we explored in this chapter doesn't just cause discomfort; it actively steals some of your 7 Freedoms. By using Tapping to rewire this pattern, you're not just getting rid of a problem–you're reclaiming your birthright to a full, vibrant life.

Take a moment to reflect: Which of these freedoms would open up the most for you if this pattern no longer had a hold on you?

- The freedom to experience emotions without being overwhelmed.
- The freedom to respond with wisdom instead of reacting from old wounds.
- The freedom to feel calm in situations that used to throw you.
- The freedom to access energy you didn't know you had.
- The freedom to feel at home and peaceful in your body.
- The freedom to trust yourself to handle whatever comes your way.
- The freedom to show up as your real self, not who you've been conditioned to be.

What is the first thing you would do, create, or experience with this newfound freedom?

It's Time to Stop Letting Fear Make Decisions for You

The thing is, fear is currently making your decisions for you. It's choosing your job, your relationships, your life. You think you're playing it safe, but you're just playing small. What if the thing you're most afraid of has already happened—you've let fear run your life?

And that fear, the one that's made decisions for you, limited your choices, exhausted your energy, what if that's just outdated programming that can be updated?

Not managed. Not endured. Not gradually weakened over years of uncomfortable practice.

THE DATA: Fears by the Numbers

When users complete sessions in The Tapping Solution App, they rate their intensity from 0 to 10 before and after the Tapping meditations.

When we analyzed usage patterns across 32 million sessions in The Tapping Solution App, some striking patterns emerged about the results people get when they practice Tapping for different fears:

- Fear of flying: 43 percent average reduction in pre-flight anxiety
- Fear of public speaking: 50 percent average reduction in pre-event anxiety
- Fear of the dentist: 41 percent average reduction in pre-appointment anxiety
- Claustrophobia: 35 percent average reduction in in-the-moment distress

One 2022 study on Tapping for fear of flying led to a 50 percent decrease in fear scores.[11]

Other studies have found that even just one Tapping session can significantly reduce specific fears—with improvements that last months and even years after the Tapping session.[12]

Now, 50 percent is significant. Moving from feeling fear at a level 8 to fear at a level 4 is the difference between getting on the plane to your dream vacation, or not. It's the difference between presenting to your client and landing the deal, or not. It's the difference between going after your dreams and living your life to the fullest, or not.

Updated. Reprogrammed. Rewired.

The woman at the airport discovered she wasn't destined to be "someone who can't fly." She was someone stuck in a fear-based Reactive Loop, running old programming that could be changed in 10 minutes once she hit that Choice Point at the gate.

Octavia learned she wasn't "the woman afraid of dogs." She was someone whose protective system had overcorrected and could be recalibrated.

Christian realized he wasn't "naturally anxious as a passenger." He was running a 25-year-old program based on a single incident that no longer applied, keeping him stuck in a Familiarity Trap.

What old programming are you running? What patterns have convinced you "this is just how I am"?

Here's the truth: How you've always been is not how you have to stay.

YOUR "NO" LIST: THE PRICE OF FEAR

Let's get brutally honest about the cost of fear in *your* life.

Part 1: The "No" List

Take a moment and make a list (in your mind or on paper) that you've said no to because of fear. Job opportunities? Trips? Relationships? Love? How long is that list?

Here are a few common fears and the "no's" they can create in our lives.

- **Fear of the dentist, the doctor, needles, etc.:** This means saying no to preventative care, to addressing a health concern, or to feeling comfortable during a necessary procedure.
- **Fear of animals:** This can mean saying no to visiting a friend's house, to going for a walk in the park, or to your family's dream of getting a puppy.
- **Fear of heights, small spaces, or water:** This means saying no to hiking with a beautiful view, to taking an elevator to a rooftop party, or to enjoying a boat ride with your family.
- **Fear of driving:** This means saying no to job opportunities in a neighboring town, to visiting family who live far away, or to the simple freedom of running your own errands.
- **Fear of social situations:** This means saying no to parties, to networking events that could advance your career, or to the wedding of someone you love.
- **Fear of failure:** This might mean saying no to applying for that dream job, starting the business you've always imagined, writing that book, making that art, or even learning a new skill.
- **Fear of rejection:** This could look like saying no to asking for a raise, pitching a new client, or sharing your true opinion with a group of friends.

- **Fear of conflict:** This often means saying no to setting a necessary boundary with a family member, disagreeing with your boss, or choosing to make a decision for yourself that might disrupt the peace.
- **Fear of public speaking:** This might mean saying no to giving a toast at a wedding, taking on a leadership role, or even just speaking up in a meeting.

Part 2: What is the cost of those "no's"?

Look at one of the most significant items on your list. Let's feel the weight of it for a moment.

- Ask yourself: "What has been the true cost of avoiding this? Not just the missed event, but the missed memories, the missed confidence, the missed joy?"
- Complete this sentence: "Because of this fear, a part of me has never been able to . . ."

Part 3: What would happen without the fear?

This is the most important part. I want you to close your eyes. Imagine for a moment that this fear is just . . . gone. You are free.

- **What is the very first thing you do?** Don't think about it, just feel it. Picture the scene in vivid detail. Where are you? Who are you with? What are you wearing?
- **What does it feel like in your body to be doing this?** Is there a lightness in your chest? A sense of excitement in your stomach? A feeling of peace in your shoulders? Connect with that physical sensation of freedom.
- **What choices do you now have that you didn't before?** With that sense of freedom, what possibilities open up? What might you choose to do next?

This vision, this feeling of possibility, it's not just a fantasy. This is the destination awaiting you when you rewire this loop.

The Freedom of New Programming

What happens when you stop being limited by old patterns?

Octavia put it perfectly: "I felt as if I had my life back again."

But it's more than getting your life back. It's discovering who you are when fear isn't programming your choices. It's finding out what becomes possible when you're not running software designed for situations that no longer exist.

The woman at the airport didn't just overcome a flying phobia. She rewired her identity from "someone who can't travel" to "someone who chooses possibility over limitation."

Christian didn't just become comfortable as a passenger. He updated his entire relationship with trust and control. The fear that had taught him he was only safe when in complete control finally released its grip, allowing him to relax into trust in other areas of his life too.

This is what's waiting for you: not just the absence of fear, but the presence of choice. Not just doing what you couldn't do before, but becoming who you really are when outdated programming stops running your life.

Your fear patterns have been loyal programs, running faithfully for years to keep you safe. But programs written for old threats don't serve your current reality.

It's time for an update. Time to install new software. Time to discover what you're capable of when you're not limited by programming that no longer serves you.

You don't have to be who you've always been. You don't have to feel what you've always felt. You don't have to be limited by patterns that were installed years ago.

You can be rewired. And it can happen faster than you ever imagined.

Ready to update your programming?

Let's tap.

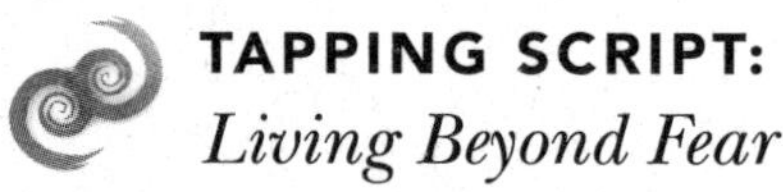

TAPPING SCRIPT: *Living Beyond Fear*

Let's take a moment to check in.

How are you feeling about the things that make you fearful or hold you back? Those situations you tend to avoid or that make your heart race? Give your overall fear level a number from 0 to 10, where 10 is "very fearful" and 0 is "completely calm."

Take a gentle breath in . . . and out.

Start tapping on the side of your hand. Repeat either in your mind or out loud.

Side of the Hand: Even though I have these fears and anxieties
that limit my life in certain ways,
I acknowledge how I feel right now.

Even though certain situations make me want to pull back,
and I wish I felt more confident,
I'm open to moving forward in a new way.

Even though I sometimes play it safe,
I'm open to expanding my comfort zone.

Eyebrow: This fear
Side of the Eye: This anxiety
Under the Eye: The way it builds in my body
Under the Nose: It leaves me feeling like I have no control
Under the Mouth: This fear has been taking me over
Collarbone: But it's safe to take my power back
Under the Arm: I acknowledge this fear's good intentions
Top of the Head: It's just trying to keep me safe

Eyebrow: As I look closer at this pattern . . .
Side of the Eye: I notice how it's been holding me back
Under the Eye: I don't need to hold on to this fear . . .
Under the Nose: and I'm here to let my mind and body know . . .
Under the Mouth: that I can ease this fear . . .
Collarbone: and still be safe
Under the Arm: I recognize any resistance . . .
Top of the Head: and I give myself the reassurance I need

Eyebrow: I am not defined by this fear
Side of the Eye: I am smart and capable
Under the Eye: I can handle more than I realize
Under the Nose: I don't have to stay limited
Under the Mouth: I turn down the volume of this fear . . .

Collarbone: so I can open up to new possibilities
Under the Arm: As I begin to quiet this fear . . .
Top of the Head: I expand my comfort zone

Eyebrow: My body is learning it is safe
Side of the Eye: I'm finding my courage
Under the Eye: Relaxing into this new confidence
Under the Nose: Feeling more ease in my body
Under the Mouth: Grounding myself in this moment
Collarbone: Relaxing my shoulders and jaw
Under the Arm: Feeling a new sense of safety
Top of the Head: I am expanding into new possibilities

Gently stop tapping and let your hands rest. Take a deep breath in . . . and let it out slowly.

Check back in with yourself now. Where's your anxiety level on that 0-to-10 scale? Notice if you feel even a little more spacious or calm.

You've just shown your nervous system that it's safe to relax. Those limitations don't have to define your life.

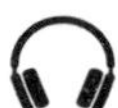

For a guided audio version of this Tapping meditation, visit www.thetappingsolution.com/rewired.

TO REMEMBER . . .

The Core Insight: *A deep-seated fear is not a permanent part of who you are; it's an outdated survival program running on repeat. But you have the power to update this software. You are no longer in the situation that created the fear, and you have the agency to teach your body it's finally safe in the here and now.*

The Practice: *Become the programmer of your own nervous system. Your practice is to acknowledge the fear and bring the old program to mind, and then use Tapping to rewire the old response. By pairing the old trigger with a new signal of calm, you are actively taking control of the wiring and rewriting the code from "danger" to "safe." That's when you discover who you are and what's possible when outdated patterns stop limiting your choices.*

CHAPTER 9

When the Past Won't Stay in the Past

Healing Old Wounds That Still Hurt

I was supposed to be in a *very* important meeting in 30 minutes. Instead, I was standing shirtless on a Manhattan sidewalk, blood on my hands, watching an ambulance pull away.

Five minutes earlier, I'd been walking to my meeting when a woman fell on the sidewalk and cut her wrist—badly—on a glass bottle she was holding that broke. Without thinking, I ran over and ripped off my gray collared polo shirt to stop the bleeding. I took the best care of her I could, wrapping my polo shirt around her wrist and calling 911. Other strangers helped; the ambulance arrived after what seemed like an eternity and whisked her away, along with my blood-soaked polo shirt, to get treated properly.

Now, with 30 minutes until my meeting and wearing nothing but jeans and dress shoes, I was shirtless. Walking down the street in the East Village in New York City shirtless is an experience I'll never forget (and maybe not surprisingly, given where I was in the world, I received fewer strange looks than one would expect)!

I walked to a coffee shop a few blocks away that happened to have some shirts on the walls, explained why I was entering the shop shirtless, and the lovely man at the counter sold me a new shirt (and was kind enough to give me a discount on it). The meeting went great, and I had a good story to open it with. The woman was safe and taken care of.

But for days afterward, my brain wouldn't let it go.

The scene played on repeat: The crashing fall. Going to help her, thinking I was just helping someone back up. Seeing how much blood there was and how big of a cut she had. Ripping off my shirt to stop the bleeding. The fall. The blood. The shirt. The fall. The blood. The shirt. My nervous system had captured the moment in high definition and wouldn't stop hitting replay.

I wasn't deeply traumatized. But my body had clearly flagged this as Important: File Under "Things That Need Processing."

The replay wouldn't stop.

This is how it works, isn't it? Sometimes it's the massive traumas that replay again and again. Sometimes it's the smaller moments our brains decide are significant enough to keep on repeat. Either way, these "Memory Replays" make us involuntary time travelers, yanked back to moments we'd rather leave behind.

I did what I knew to do: I tapped. The replay slowed, then stopped. My nervous system finally got the memo that the emergency was over.

But here's what struck me about this experience: I've been teaching Tapping for years, I know the science inside and out, and yet my brain still got stuck in that pattern.

It's a reminder that we're all wired the same way. Our nervous systems don't care about our credentials or our knowledge or our logic. They follow ancient programming that says: "This was significant. Keep replaying until processed."

So, what about when those Memory Replays have been playing for years? Decades? What about when your past doesn't just visit, but it moves in, redecorates, and refuses to leave?

The Dispatcher Who Couldn't Turn Off the Scanner

When my sister, Jessica, first spoke with Samantha, she described something we've heard from so many first responders. She'd been the rock everyone leaned on. As a 911 dispatcher, she was the calm voice in countless crises. "You're so solid," her mother would say. "Nothing rattles you."

For years, this seemed true. Samantha could handle anything: fatal car accidents, domestic violence calls, parents discovering children who'd stopped breathing. She was professional, composed, effective. Her nervous system had learned to stay absolutely steady while helping other people navigate their worst moments.

Then she left dispatching. Her son went back to school. Life slowed down.

That's when all hell broke loose.

"It was like my brain suddenly realized it was safe to process everything I'd heard," Samantha told Jessica. "And it decided to process it all at once."

She couldn't go to the mall without mapping escape routes. Couldn't see a playground without imagining which child might get hurt. The hypervigilance that had made her an excellent dispatcher now made regular life unbearable. Her brain stayed tuned to the emergency frequency even though she'd turned in her headset years ago.

Sleep became her enemy. Every time she closed her eyes, her brain served up a highlight reel of every traumatic call she'd ever taken. She'd wake at 3 A.M., heart pounding, responding to emergencies that had happened five years earlier.

This is the particular cruelty of trauma: It doesn't respect retirement. It doesn't care that you've moved on, changed careers, tried to build a different life. Your nervous system remains loyal to old programming, playing by rules that no longer apply.

Samantha's hypervigilance was a specific type of Reactive Loop. Her nervous system had learned that constant scanning for danger = survival. Even though she'd left dispatching, her amygdala hadn't gotten the memo. It was still running the Emergency Dispatcher program 24/7, flooding her system with stress hormones and keeping her threat-detection system on maximum sensitivity.

PAUSE *and* REFLECT: IDENTIFYING YOUR OWN MEMORY REPLAYS

Take a moment right now. What's one memory that your brain likes to replay uninvited? Maybe it's not as dramatic as a sidewalk emergency—maybe it's:

- That conversation that went badly
- The mistake you made at work
- The relationship that ended painfully
- The moment you felt humiliated

Notice: How often does this memory visit you? Daily? Weekly? When you're trying to sleep?

Rate the intensity: On a scale of 0 to 10, how much does this memory still affect you when it shows up?

The Delayed Reaction: When Safety Becomes Dangerous

Here's something I wish everyone understood: Often, trauma symptoms don't appear until you're finally safe.

I've seen this pattern hundreds of times. Veterans come home and *then* fall apart. First responders retire and *then* can't function. Abuse survivors escape and *then* struggle more than when they were in danger.

When you're in survival mode, your nervous system suppresses anything that might interfere with keeping you alive. Processing emotions? Luxury. Feeling your feelings? Can't afford it. Your system locks everything in a vault marked "Deal With Later."

This is the cruelest form of the Familiarity Trap: Your nervous system thinks constant hypervigilance is "safer" than processing and releasing.

Then you actually get safe. And your nervous system, helpful as ever, says: "Oh good! Now we're in a place where we can finally process all this!" And proceeds to dump 20 years of suppressed trauma on you on a casual Thursday afternoon.

Samantha discovered this the hard way. The very safety she'd worked so hard to create became the condition that allowed her trauma to surface. The rock everyone had leaned on was crumbling, and she didn't understand why.

WHEN DID THINGS SHIFT FOR YOU?

Samantha's hypervigilance kicked in after she left dispatching. Think about your own life:

- When did you first notice yourself being "on guard" all the time?
- Was there a specific period when life felt overwhelming?
- Did symptoms appear during a "safe" time, catching you off guard?

Write down or mentally note: What was happening in your life when these patterns started? Sometimes identifying the timing helps us understand why our nervous system made the choices it did.

The Night Everything Changed

When Samantha told Jessica what happened next, she got goose bumps.

Desperate for sleep, she found our app and clicked on something called "Micro Boost of Safety." This is a super quick Tapping session that's just three minutes long. She was skeptical about Tapping but exhausted enough to try anything.

"It was a game changer," she told me, and the wonder was still in her voice. "I could actually fall asleep. And stay asleep."

Every night, Samantha hit the same **Choice Point**: Surrender to the familiar replay of traumatic calls or interrupt the pattern with Tapping.

Tap, tap, tap. Teaching her nervous system: You're safe now. The emergency is over. You can rest. Night after night, she chose to Recognize the loop starting, Interrupt it with Tapping, and slowly Rewire her nervous system's default from "the world is dangerous" to "I am safe now."

Then one night, she forgot to do the Tapping.

To her surprise, she still slept great that night. That's when she knew the rewiring was complete.

She realized she had done it. She had gotten her body to a place that it actually felt safe. She didn't need to do the nightly Tapping anymore, because her body had actually rewired and now knew it was safe to sleep.

This is exactly what we hope for, not that people need to tap forever, but that Tapping rewires the system so thoroughly that the old patterns simply stop running. For good.

Samantha's nervous system updated its software. The emergency broadcast system finally switched off.

And yours can too.

What would change if you could actually rest with ease? If you could actually live without being on guard?

The Inferno That Wouldn't Stop Burning

Millie's e-mail arrived in my inbox a few years after her building burned down. Even reading it, I could feel the intensity of that night.

At 4 A.M. on December 22, she woke to the smell of smoke. Within minutes, she was pounding on doors, evacuating neighbors. Everyone got out in time, but just minutes later, the entire building was in flames.

Everyone survived. Miraculous, given how fast the fire spread. But Millie's nervous system didn't get the memo that the crisis had passed.

"I kept reliving it," she wrote. "The sounds, the smells, and the sheer panic."

A psychiatrist friend, and I love that it was a psychiatrist who recommended this, introduced her to Tapping. She did two sessions with her friend, and noticed progress, but felt like she needed to do more Tapping and her friend was busy. So she turned to our free guided "Releasing Anxiety" Tapping meditation.

"It became my lifeline," Millie explained. "Not just for the trauma, but for sleep, anxiety, focus—everything. Two years later, I still use it. Some people have security blankets. I have Tapping."

That last line made me smile. But it also points to something profound: When we give people tools to regulate their own nervous systems, we give them back their power. Millie doesn't need to wait for a therapy appointment or a prescription refill. She has what she needs, literally at her fingertips.

What if you had that kind of power in your pocket?

25 Years of Proof

Of all the stories that have come through our community, Windy's might be the one that shows most powerfully what's possible when we rewire trauma responses.

Twenty-five years. That's how long she lived with domestic violence and emotional abuse. When she finally escaped in 2020, she thought the hard part was over.

She was wrong.

"I was having flashbacks and night terrors," she shared with me. "I would wake multiple times a night in terror, unable to remember what year it was or where I was. It was terrifying."

Her therapist kept suggesting Tapping for these 2 A.M. wake-ups. Finally, in desperation, Windy tried it.

"One night at 2 A.M. when I woke in a sweat of terror, I went into the bathroom and sat and began to tap. After about an hour I was able to return to sleep. Each time I woke, I tapped again. On night three I was able to go back to sleep after 15 minutes of Tapping."

But here's where Windy's story becomes remarkable, and why I knew I had to share it with you. She didn't just use Tapping for the night terrors. She used it to navigate a volatile divorce, court appearances, litigation. While her ex-husband tried to trigger her old trauma responses, she tapped under desks, in bathroom stalls, during court breaks.

"Tapping helped me to show up in a regulated state," she said. "It helped me defend myself without being pulled away by the somatic responses."

Windy's story is a remarkable one. Twenty-five years of programming, rewired. A nervous system that had only known danger learning safety. A woman discovering she could face her abuser in court without being pulled back into old patterns.

This is what we mean by rewiring. Not erasing the past; Windy's experiences still happened. But changing how her nervous system responds to triggers. Updating the software so the past stops hijacking the present.

The Orphans Who Stopped Reliving Genocide

Sometimes I hesitate to share this next study because the numbers seem impossible. But it's been published, peer-reviewed, and the implications are staggering.

Researchers worked with 50 orphaned teenagers in Rwanda who had survived the genocide. These young people had severe PTSD for over a decade. They'd tried various interventions with limited success.

The research team provided one session—ONE SESSION—of Tapping (specifically, they used Thought Field Therapy, or TFT, the parent technique to EFT Tapping).

Before the session: 100 percent of the children met criteria for PTSD according to caregiver reports. After the session: Only 6 percent still met criteria.[13]

Even a year later, the improvements held.

I need to be clear: This needs replication. There was no control group. Cultural factors could be at play. But still . . . from 100 percent to 6 percent? In one session? For trauma that had persisted for over a decade?

When I read studies like this, I think about what we're really seeing. Not just symptom reduction, but nervous systems remembering how to find peace. Not just coping with trauma, but genuinely metabolizing it.

THE VELOCITY PRINCIPLE

When we hear stories or studies like these, we're likely to wonder: How can a decade of pain be resolved so quickly? It's because our healing doesn't operate on a linear, one-to-one timeline with our suffering. This is governed by a powerful truth that offers incredible hope, a concept we call the **Velocity Principle**.

THE RULE:
The duration of the problem does not dictate the duration of the healing.

We are conditioned to believe that if we have suffered for 20 years, it will take another 20 years to heal. This single belief keeps millions of people stuck, feeling that the path to healing is too long and arduous to even begin.

But when you use a tool that speaks directly to the nervous system and updates the neurological source code–the original memory–transformation can be rapid and permanent. The stories in this chapter, from Windy's 25 years of struggle to the Rwandan teens' decade of PTSD, are not exceptions to the rule. They *are* the rule. When you have the right key, a lock that has been rusted shut for years can open in an instant.

Your Nervous System's Emergency Broadcast System

I'm going to get technical for a moment, because understanding the mechanism makes what can seem like a miracle make perfect, logical sense.

When trauma happens, your amygdala (remember, that's your brain's alarm system) essentially gets stuck in the "on" position. It keeps broadcasting "DANGER! DANGER!" even when the danger has passed.

Tapping speaks directly to the amygdala through the body. Those acupoints we tap on? They send calming signals through the same pathways that are carrying the alarm signals. It's like finally finding the off switch for an alarm that's been blaring for years.

The research backs this up. Studies show:

- 90 percent of veterans with PTSD no longer met criteria after just six Tapping sessions
- Cortisol levels drop by up to 43 percent after single sessions
- VA clinics now offer Tapping to veterans dealing with PTSD

YOUR ALARM SYSTEM ASSESSMENT

Your amygdala might be stuck in the "on" position if you experience:

- ❑ Jumping at sudden noises
- ❑ Constant scanning for danger
- ❑ Physical tension you can't release
- ❑ Difficulty trusting that you're safe
- ❑ Feeling like something bad is about to happen
- ❑ Sleep issues
- ❑ Avoiding things that are logically safe but make you feel on edge
- ❑ Feeling exhausted but wired

How many did you check? Each checkmark is your nervous system saying, "I'm still not sure we're safe."

The Truth About Trauma

Here's what 20 years of this work has taught me: Trauma isn't what happened to you. Trauma is what your nervous system is still doing about what happened to you.

The event is over. The replay is the problem.

The fire is out. The smoke alarm is still screaming. The danger has passed. But the body hasn't gotten the update.

This isn't minimizing what happened. Your experiences were real. Your pain is valid. Your struggles make perfect sense.

There's a line from the TV show *True Detective*: "Time is a flat circle." For trauma survivors, this isn't philosophy; it's daily reality. The past doesn't feel past. It feels perpetually present.

But here's what I've witnessed thousands of times: people breaking free from that circle. The past becoming actually the past. The body learning that the emergency really is over.

This is the radical, hope-filled truth—your nervous system's response can change. The Mental Replays can stop. The alarm can finally switch off.

Not through thinking your way out (you've tried that). Not through time alone (you've waited). Not through pretending it didn't matter (it did).

But through giving your body the direct experience of safety while the memory is active. Through tapping while the memory plays, teaching your system: "This is a memory, not a current threat."

THE COST CALCULATOR

Let's get real about what these Mental Replays are costing you:

Energy: What percentage of your mental energy goes to managing old pain? 10 percent? 50 percent? 90 percent?

Relationships: How is the past affecting your ability to connect? Are you:

- Keeping people at arm's length?
- Overreacting to small triggers?
- Unable to be fully present?

Life Choices: What are you *not* doing because the past won't let go?

- Career moves you're avoiding?
- Relationships you won't pursue?
- Dreams you've shelved?

The Bottom Line: If the past wasn't taking up so much space, what would you do with all that freed-up energy, attention, and courage?

Your Past's Eviction Notice

As we close this chapter, I want to leave you with this:

Your past has had a good run. It's been running your sleep, your relationships, your sense of safety in the world. It's been a terrible tenant—never paying rent, making too much noise, refusing to leave.

So, it's time for the eviction notice.

You don't have to live like this. Samantha sleeps through the night now. Millie can smell smoke from a neighbor's fireplace without panicking. Windy faced her abuser in court with a regulated nervous system. Thousands of people have discovered their past can finally become past tense.

And it's your turn to break free from the past. It's your turn to escape this particular Familiarity Trap of yesteryear.

Every time you tap while a memory surfaces, you're not just processing, you're rewiring. You're taking that old Reactive Loop (this memory = current danger) and creating a new Rewired Response (this memory = something that already happened). Each tap at that Choice Point teaches your nervous system to respond differently.

Every session is a step toward freedom. Every round is your nervous system learning "This already happened. We survived. We're safe now." Every tap is proof that change is possible.

The time traveler's curse can be broken. The emergency broadcast can finally end. The past can stop colonizing your present. Every tap is you choosing at that Choice Point to Recognize the old loop, Interrupt it, and Rewire your nervous system for the present moment, where you're actually safe.

Ready to serve that eviction notice?

Let's tap.

RECLAIMING *Your* FREEDOMS

The pattern we explored in this chapter doesn't just cause discomfort; it actively steals some of your 7 Freedoms. By using Tapping to rewire this pattern, you're not just getting rid of a problem–you're reclaiming your birthright to a full, vibrant life.

Take a moment to reflect: Which of these freedoms would open up the most for you if this pattern no longer had a hold on you?

- The freedom to experience emotions without being overwhelmed.
- The freedom to respond with wisdom instead of reacting from old wounds.
- The freedom to feel calm in situations that used to throw you.
- The freedom to access energy you didn't know you had.
- The freedom to feel at home and peaceful in your body.
- The freedom to trust yourself to handle whatever comes your way.
- The freedom to show up as your real self, not who you've been conditioned to be.

What is the first thing you would do, create, or experience with this newfound freedom?

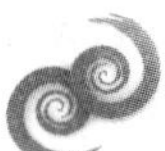

TAPPING SCRIPT:
Release the Charge of Memory Replays

Let's check in.

We all have memories that sometimes pop up uninvited—maybe an embarrassing moment, a difficult conversation, something we wish had gone differently, or painful memories. As you read the chapter, did a particular memory come up? Is there a memory that you come back to again and again?

Important note: This is not intended to be deep trauma work. For this experience, choose a memory that is uncomfortable, but not overwhelming.

Bring your chosen memory to mind now, and give the stress or anxiety you feel a number from 0 to 10, where 10 is "I feel very anxious" and 0 is "I feel at ease."

Take a gentle breath in . . . and out.

Start tapping on the side of your hand. Repeat either in your mind or out loud.

Side of the Hand: Even though this memory keeps playing in my mind, I choose to breathe deeply now.

Even though I keep thinking about what happened, I am open to finding more ease.

Even though part of me is still stuck in that moment, I'm ready to take my power back.

Eyebrow: This memory on repeat
Side of the Eye: My mind won't let it go
Under the Eye: Analyzing every detail
Under the Nose: Trying to figure out what went wrong . . .
Under the Mouth: and what it all means
Collarbone: But I can't change what happened
Under the Arm: I acknowledge all these feelings
Top of the Head: I'm open to transforming this memory

Eyebrow: I can reflect on this memory from a distance
Side of the Eye: Remembering that was then . . .

Under the Eye: and this is now
Under the Nose: It's safe for my body to relax
Under the Mouth: The danger has passed
Collarbone: I'm growing from this experience . . .
Under the Arm: and realizing my strength
Top of the Head: Allowing this memory to lose some of its power

Eyebrow: If I notice this memory playing . . .
Side of the Eye: I can catch the pattern
Under the Eye: It's an invitation to check in with myself . . .
Under the Nose: and remind myself that I am safe now
Under the Mouth: I'm creating a new pattern
Collarbone: One of safety
Under the Arm: I know how to take care of myself . . .
Top of the Head: and find my way back to the present moment

Eyebrow: I choose to be in the here and now . . .
Side of the Eye: where I am safe
Under the Eye: I can come back here again and again
Under the Nose: Letting old stories rest
Under the Mouth: My body can let down its guard
Collarbone: I'm safe in this moment
Under the Arm: Making room for new possibilities
Top of the Head: Feeling safe and hopeful

Gently stop tapping and let your hands rest. Take a deep breath in . . . and let it out slowly.

Check back in with yourself now. Allow yourself to think back on that memory. Do you still feel anxiety, or more ease? Give your stress a new number on the 0 to 10 scale.

You've just begun teaching your nervous system that the past is truly past. You're safe to be present now.

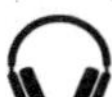

For a guided audio version of this Tapping meditation, visit www.thetappingsolution.com/rewired.

To Remember . . .

The Core Insight: *When a painful memory intrudes on your present, it is your nervous system's attempt to process an experience that it couldn't handle in the past. It's an open loop seeking completion. The hopeful truth is that this replay is an invitation. You have the agency to finally give that memory the resolution it's been seeking.*

The Practice: *When a memory or a painful feeling from the past resurfaces, see it as an opportunity to finally close the loop. Your practice is to meet these echoes from the past with a new, calming response. Instead of pushing it away or being consumed by it, tap through it. This allows you to teach your nervous system that you are safe now, and that the past truly is in the past—freeing you up to be truly present in the here and now.*

CHAPTER 10

When You Can't Find Motivation

Tapping Into Energy and Flow

It's 7:23 A.M. and you're having that familiar internal conversation. You know the one.

"Time to get up," you tell yourself. "But it's so comfortable here," you respond. "You have things to do." "They can wait." "You'll feel better once you start." "Doubt it."

This debate continues while your phone buzzes with notifications about all the life you're supposed to be living. Your to-do list grows. Your anxiety builds. Your motivation remains exactly where it was: nowhere to be found.

It's like your get-up-and-go got up and went without you.

Welcome to the motivation paradox: The more you need it, the less you have it. The more you chase it, the faster it runs. The more you beat yourself up about not having it, the deeper it burrows into hiding.

But what if I told you that your lack of motivation isn't a character flaw? What if it's not laziness, weakness, or proof that you're broken?

What if it's just your nervous system stuck in a very specific Reactive Loop—one that can be interrupted, rewired, and transformed?

The MS Warrior Who Found Her Spark

Amee had every reason to stay in bed. Multiple sclerosis. Chronic low energy. A list of housework that felt like climbing Everest in flip-flops.

"I kept putting it off," she told me, and I could hear the frustration in her message. This wasn't laziness talking; this was someone whose body was fighting against her every day.

But one morning, before even getting out of bed, Amee tried something different. She tapped along to a Tapping meditation called "Motivate Me to Have a Productive Day."

What happened next still makes me grin:

"I got through my list with ease! And more! Goodness me! And to think I have MS and low energy! What on earth happened to me today? Even my husband said I should slow down. I've been on such a high all day and . . . I'm so chuffed with what I have achieved!"

Let's pause here. A woman with a chronic illness that attacks her energy systems didn't just complete her to-do list. She exceeded it so thoroughly that her husband, who presumably knows her limits better than anyone, told her to slow down.

She went from "can't get out of bed" to "on such a high" all in one morning.

How?

Through the REWIRED process in action: She Recognized her lack-of-motivation loop, Interrupted it with Tapping, and Rewired her nervous system's response.

The Motivation Myth We Need to Destroy

Here's what nobody tells you about motivation: You don't need to feel it to have it.

Okay, okay, but what do I mean by that?

We've been sold this idea that motivation is a feeling—a warm, energized, "Let's do this!" sensation. That we need to *feel* motivated before we can *act* motivated. That's like saying you need to feel strong before you can lift weights or feel smart before you can learn something new.

Motivation isn't a feeling. It's a state of nervous system readiness.

Let me break down what's actually happening in your body when you "can't find motivation."

1. **The Dopamine Drought:** Your brain's reward system runs on dopamine, the "Let's do this!" chemical. But when stress hormones flood your system, they block dopamine receptors. It's like putting gum in a lock; the key (dopamine) can't get in to unlock your motivation. No wonder nothing feels worth doing.
2. **The Prefrontal Shutdown:** Under stress, blood flow diverts away from your prefrontal cortex (your brain's CEO) to your survival centers. You lose access to the part of your brain that knows how to plan, prioritize, and take action. It's like trying to run a company when the CEO's office has no power.
3. **The Norepinephrine Paradox:** Stress triggers norepinephrine, which should energize you. But in chronic stress, your receptors become resistant. You're flooded with "go" chemicals but can't access their energy, like a car with the accelerator stuck but the transmission in neutral.
4. **The Mitochondrial Mutiny:** Your cellular power plants (mitochondria) can reduce energy production by up to 50 percent when under stress. They're rationing power because they think you're in crisis mode. Every task feels exhausting because you're running on emergency backup power.
5. **The GABA Blockade:** GABA (gamma-aminobutyric acid) is your brain's brake pedal; it helps you feel calm and focused. But chronic stress depletes GABA, leaving you anxious and scattered. Without GABA, your brain can't filter out distractions or settle into productive flow.

Maybe you recognize these sensations:

- **The Fog:** Your mind goes blank when you try to think about the task. Simple planning feels impossibly complex. You can't figure out where to start.
- **The Weight:** Your body feels physically heavy, like gravity got turned up. Getting off the couch requires superhuman effort. Your limbs feel like lead.
- **The Void:** Nothing sounds appealing. Things you usually enjoy feel flat and colorless. It's not sadness exactly—it's the absence of want.

- **The Wall:** There's an invisible barrier between you and action. You can see what needs to be done, but you can't make yourself move toward it. It's like trying to push through thick glass.
- **The Drain:** Just thinking about the task exhausts you. You feel tired before you've done anything, because your nervous system is already burning energy in the freeze response.

When Amee tapped that morning, she wasn't manufacturing fake enthusiasm. She wasn't giving herself a pep talk. She was shifting her nervous system from "protection mode" to "possibility mode."

And here's the kicker: When your nervous system shifts, motivation isn't something you need to find. It's something that finds you.

Your natural drive to engage with life, to complete tasks, to create and contribute; it's all there under the stress response. You don't need to generate it. You need to stop suppressing it.

The Perfectionism Trap That Kills Motivation

Jessica once worked with a woman who couldn't find motivation to lose weight, no matter how much she wanted to make the change for her health.

During their session, the woman shared something her father used to say: "Go big or go home." He'd meant it to be supportive, encouraging her to aim high. But for her, it had become a paralyzing perfectionism trap: Do it perfectly or don't do it at all.

"We don't give ourselves grace to figure things out, to fail, to learn," Jessica observes. "We think we need to get it right the first time, and that impossible standard kills motivation before we even begin."

This is a classic Reactive Loop where the fear of imperfection triggers a "freeze" state.

But the antidote to all of that is learning it's okay if you don't have it all figured out. It's okay if it doesn't go perfectly the first time. We need to allow ourselves to take life a little less serious and allow ourselves to fail once in a while.

As Arianna Huffington once told Jessica in an interview: "Failure is not the opposite of success; it's part of it."

If you look at failure as just part of the course, you stay on the course.

Your motivation isn't missing because you're lazy. It's missing because you're terrified of not getting it right. And that fear keeps you stuck in the familiar pattern of not trying at all.

One of the greatest freedoms you will gain from this book is the freedom to be imperfect. The freedom to take life a little less seriously, and enjoy the ups and downs along the way. When you can tap away the fear of "not getting it right," your motivation to simply try and move forward comes roaring back to life.

The Procrastination Loop (And Why Your Brain Loves It)

Let me map out what's really happening when motivation goes missing:

1. **The Freeze State:** Your nervous system perceives some threat in the task ahead. Maybe it's fear of failure, fear of success, or just fear of the effort required. Your system responds by going into a mild freeze state.
2. **The Protection Pattern:** Procrastination isn't laziness—it's protection. Your brain is trying to keep you safe from whatever threat it perceives in that task. Can't fail if you don't try, right? This is your nervous system's Familiarity Trap at work, choosing the known discomfort of procrastination over the unknown risks of action.
3. **The Energy Drain:** Fighting against this protection pattern burns massive energy. You're not just not doing the thing, you're actively wrestling with not doing the thing. It's exhausting.
4. **The Shame Spiral:** Now you feel bad about procrastinating, which activates more stress, which triggers more protection, which drains more energy . . . see the loop?

This is why willpower doesn't work. You're trying to override a protection mechanism with force. It's like trying to open a door by pushing harder when it opens by pulling.

This entire Reactive Loop is a **Familiarity Trap** masterpiece. Your brain has gotten so good at this pattern—Freeze, Protect, Drain, Shame, Repeat—that it runs automatically. It's exhausting and self-defeating, but it's familiar. And that familiarity feels safer than the uncertainty of actually doing the thing.

Every task you avoid is a **Choice Point** where your nervous system chooses the familiar (procrastination) over the possible (action). Tapping interrupts this at the source, teaching your system: "We don't have to be who we've always been. We can be someone who just . . . gets things done."

WHERE DO YOU STRUGGLE MOST WITH MOTIVATION?

What area of your life do you have a hard time getting started? Where do you feel lack of energy? Where do you drag your feet?

- Exercise?
- Work?
- Working on a passion project?
- House projects?
- Clearing clutter or organizing?
- Doing the dishes?

When Your Morning Sets the Tone for Everything

Here's a scene from Alex's life a few years ago that might be familiar to some of you: Three kids under four years old. Chaos from the moment his feet hit the floor. Breakfast negotiations. Lost shoes. Sibling battles. The morning scramble that leaves every parent feeling like they've already run a marathon by 8 A.M.

"When they're finally off to school," he described, "you're supposed to just . . . switch gears and be productive all of a sudden."

But your nervous system doesn't work like that. You can't go from battlefield commander to focused creative in the time it takes to close the front door.

This is where traditional productivity advice completely fails. It assumes you're starting from neutral. Like you're some sort of robot who can perfectly compartmentalize and dive into deep work at the drop of a hat.

The reality? Most of us carry that morning frenzy (and even residue leftover from yesterday) straight into our workday. We sit at our desks with our shoulders still tensed from rushing, our minds still racing from the morning's mini-dramas, our patience already depleted from negotiations about wearing socks.

Alex learned this the hard way. He'd drop the kids off and rush to his desk, determined to be productive. But he'd find himself staring at his computer, unable to focus, getting frustrated with himself for "wasting time."

Then he realized: It wasn't just wasting time. He was trying to work while his nervous system was still in parental-crisis mode.

THE LAW OF THE MISGUIDED PROTECTOR

To truly break this cycle, we have to change our relationship with the part of us that procrastinates. Instead of seeing it as a lazy enemy, we need to understand its true motive. This is a fundamental law for compassionate change:

THE RULE:
There are no "bad" parts of you, only protective parts running outdated software.

Your procrastination isn't a character flaw; it's a misguided bodyguard trying to keep you safe based on past threats. It's the part of you that learned, "If I don't hand in the report, I can't be judged for it," or "If I don't start the project, I can't fail."

Instead of asking, "What's wrong with me?" ask, "How is this pattern trying to protect me?" The goal isn't to eliminate this protective part, but to update its job description. With Tapping, you can gently inform that bodyguard that you're safe now, and you have better tools for handling challenges than simple avoidance.

What Actually Gets in Our Way

We've all had this experience. One day you get a hundred things done in 2 focused hours, another you barely check anything off the to-do list in a long, 10-hour day.

The difference? It has nothing to do with time management.

"When I can't motivate myself to do something, I don't think, 'Why can't I motivate myself?'" Alex says. "I think to myself, 'What is actually getting in the way?'"

As it turns out, our emotions, our thoughts, they are what truly impact our ability to just start, to just do things, to make progress on whatever it is we are trying to work on—whether that be work or cleaning the house or writing a book or exercising—whatever it may be.

"The difference between a day where you feel productive and a day where you feel like you got nothing done isn't about having better willpower," Alex told me. "It's about clearing the emotional obstacles before they turn into procrastination."

Research shows that unprocessed emotions create what neuroscientists call "cognitive load," which takes up precious bandwidth in your working memory. It's like trying to run complex software while 17 other programs are running in the background.

The Morning Ritual That Actually Works

Alex has tuned in to something about motivation that most productivity gurus miss entirely: The problem isn't your morning routine. It's what you're carrying into it.

For years, he watched high achievers (including himself) follow elaborate morning rituals—meditation, journaling, exercise, cold plunges, a protein smoothie—only to hit their desk and freeze. All that optimization, and they still couldn't start the work that mattered.

Then he noticed something. The days when he accomplished the most weren't the days with perfect routines. They were the days when he dealt with his emotional static first.

Now his morning practice looks different. Instead of trying to optimize himself into productivity, he asks himself deceptively simple questions.

"What do I actually want to accomplish today?" Then the real question: "What is likely to get in the way of that? What emotions or mental roadblocks could hold me back from accomplishing what I want?"

Maybe it's anxiety about a difficult conversation. Maybe it's overwhelm from yesterday's unfinished tasks. Maybe it's resentment about having to do something he doesn't want to do.

Then—and here's the key—he taps on whatever comes up. Before opening his e-mail inbox. Before checking his to-do list. Before the day has a chance to hijack his nervous system.

"Most people approach their day like a pilot who runs onto the plane late, already in crisis mode and just jumping into action," Alex says. "But if you're taking a flight, would you want a pilot that just runs straight onto the plane and takes off immediately? No. You'd want them to get settled, to calmly check their instruments, to do whatever they need to do to feel prepared and ready for the flight ahead."

When you clear the emotional debris before you start, motivation isn't something you need to manufacture. It's just there, waiting underneath the static.

WHAT GETS IN YOUR WAY MOST OFTEN?

When you find yourself procrastinating, or feeling low motivation to do something, what do you think is actually underneath that?

Pick one thing you've been avoiding. Let's dig deeper through the layers of what's really going on:

1. First layer: "I don't feel like it"
2. Dig deeper: What are you afraid will happen if you do it?
3. Deeper still: What are you afraid will happen if you ***don't*** do it?
4. The core: What does this avoidance protect you from feeling? Which of these feel like the true roadblock?
    - Overwhelm about how much you have to do
    - Fear of not being able to do it well
    - Worry about something else going on in your life
    - Stress about what you didn't get done yesterday
    - Guilt about other things you think you should be doing instead
    - Anxiety over what people will think when you finish the thing
    - Confusion about where to start

The Missing Piece

Rena nailed it in her message to us: "Tapping is *THE* missing piece for those of us who are stuck . . . wanting to make changes and life improvements, but unable to figure out the roadblocks holding us back."

The missing piece isn't more motivation. It's not better habits. It's not a new planner or productivity system.

The missing piece is interrupting these Reactive Loops at the nervous system level—addressing the actual neurological patterns that create motivational paralysis.

When your system feels safe, energy flows. When energy flows, action becomes natural. When action becomes natural, motivation is irrelevant.

You don't need to feel motivated to brush your teeth, do you? You just do it. That's what happens when an action isn't triggering your protection patterns.

Your Motivation Style

Through analyzing millions of Tapping sessions, we've identified five distinct patterns of "stuck." Knowing yours helps you tap more effectively.

Read these and see which one makes you say, "Ouch, that's me."

Each of these represents a different type of motivation-specific Reactive Loop:

1. **The Perfectionist Freeze:** You can't start because you might not do it perfectly. Your nervous system treats imperfection as a threat, so it keeps you safely inactive.
2. **The Overwhelm Overflow:** There's so much to do that your system shorts out. Like a computer with too many programs running, you freeze rather than risk crashing.
3. **The Purpose Void:** You can't find motivation because you can't find meaning. Your nervous system won't mobilize energy for things that don't matter.
4. **The Energy Vampire:** Something or someone is draining your reserves faster than you can refill them. You have motivation but no fuel.
5. **The Success Phobia:** You're motivated until you get close to achievement, then your system hits the brakes. Success means change, and change means danger.

Which one sounds familiar? Maybe several? That's normal—we're complex beings with complex protection patterns.

YOUR TURN TO REFLECT

1. Which one or two of these patterns are running your life?
2. Think of a particular thing you're avoiding. How does your style show up? (e.g., "I'm in a 'Perfectionist Freeze' about updating my resume," or "I'm in 'Overwhelm Overflow' about cleaning the garage.")
3. What has this pattern cost you? A promotion? Peace of mind? The joy of a clean space? The satisfaction of finishing a project?

The Productivity Trap

Before we tap, I need to address something: This chapter isn't about turning you into a productivity machine. It's not about doing more, achieving more, or pushing harder.

It's about removing the blocks between you and your natural capacity for engaged action.

Some days, that might look like Amee's housework marathon. Other days, it might look like finally having the motivation to read a book, call a friend, or take a walk.

The goal isn't maximum productivity. The goal is alignment between what you want to do and what you're able to do.

What if success isn't about doing more, but about doing the things that are important to you without the internal battle?

Why Everything Changes When the Block Lifts

When motivation returns (real motivation, not the forced kind), people describe it the same way:

"It was effortless."

"I just found myself doing it."

"I forgot it was supposed to be hard."

"I actually enjoyed it."

This is what happens when you're not fighting your own nervous system. Energy that was being used for internal battle becomes available for external action.

But here's the beautiful paradox: Often, when the pressure lifts, when you stop forcing, when your system feels safe . . . that's when you naturally do more than you ever could through force.

Amee didn't plan to become a high achiever that day. She just wanted to get through her basic housework. But when her system shifted from protection to possibility, her natural capacity emerged.

RECLAIMING *Your* FREEDOMS

The pattern we explored in this chapter doesn't just cause discomfort; it actively steals some of your 7 Freedoms. By using Tapping to rewire this pattern, you're not just getting rid of a problem—you're reclaiming your birthright to a full, vibrant life.

Take a moment to reflect: Which of these freedoms would open up the most for you if this pattern no longer had a hold on you?

- The freedom to experience emotions without being overwhelmed.
- The freedom to respond with wisdom instead of reacting from old wounds.
- The freedom to feel calm in situations that used to throw you.
- The freedom to access energy you didn't know you had.
- The freedom to feel at home and peaceful in your body.
- The freedom to trust yourself to handle whatever comes your way.
- The freedom to show up as your real self, not who you've been conditioned to be.

What is the first thing you would do, create, or experience with this newfound freedom?

The Morning That Everything Seems Different

I want to paint you a picture of what's possible:

Tomorrow morning, your alarm goes off. But instead of the usual negotiation, the usual dread, the usual "just five more minutes" that turns into 50 . . .

You tap. Right there in bed. Just acknowledging where you are and creating space for a shift.

Maybe you tap while saying:

"Even though I don't feel like getting up and starting my day, I am safe in this moment."

"Even though I'm feeling overwhelmed at the thought of all I have to do, I choose to relax my body and mind now."

"Even though I'm not feeling motivated right now, I'm open to tackling my to-do list with peace and ease."

You continue tapping through the points, allowing yourself to acknowledge how you are feeling. Nothing fancy, just tapping.

And something loosens. The weight lifts just enough. Getting up doesn't feel like climbing Everest. It just feels a little bit easier.

You move through your morning and tasks that usually feel like pulling teeth feel . . . doable. Maybe even enjoyable.

By midday, you realize you've done more than you usually do by 5 P.M. Not through forcing. Not through motivational speeches. But through removing the block that was making everything harder than it needed to be.

This isn't an unrealistic fantasy. This is everyday life for thousands of people who've discovered what Amee discovered: When you stop fighting your nervous system and start working with it, "motivation" becomes irrelevant.

You just live. You just do. You just flow.

Returning to the Choice Point

Look around your space right now. Really, do it.

How many half-finished projects do you see? Books with bookmarks at page 47? Exercise equipment doubling as clothing racks? If you're being brutally honest with yourself, what are you putting off until "someday"? Take a moment to flag the answer in your mind, or even write it down.

Right now, in this moment, you're at a Choice Point. You can close this book and go back to the motivation chase. Back to the morning negotiations. Back to the constant battle between what you want to do and what you're able to do.

Or you can try something different. Something that sounds too simple to work but has changed everything for Amee and millions of others.

You can tap. You can interrupt the loop. You can discover what's on the other side of that block.

I'm not promising you'll become a productivity superhero overnight. I'm not saying you'll suddenly love your to-do list and get a million things done that have been sitting for years.

But I am saying that motivation isn't something you need to find. It's something you need to unleash. And it's been there all along, waiting patiently under layers of protection patterns that no longer serve you.

And this is essential if you want to step into a new version of yourself. If you want to create the life you've been longing for.

Because while you're waiting for motivation to strike, your life is passing by. Dreams are expiring. Opportunities are closing. Your "someday" pile is growing while your "actually did it" pile gathers dust.

Ready to meet the motivated version of you that's been waiting in the wings?

Let's tap.

YOUR AVOIDANCE INVENTORY

Before you tap, let's get crystal clear:

1. The thing I've been avoiding most: ___________
2. How long I've been avoiding it: ___________
3. What I'm afraid will happen if I do it: ___________
4. What I know will happen if I don't: ___________
5. Am I willing to feel different about this? Yes / No / Maybe

---

TAPPING SCRIPT: *Reigniting Your Motivation*

Let's start by checking in.

Think about something you've been putting off or can't seem to start. On a scale of 0 to 10, how stuck or unmotivated do you feel about it? 10 is completely stuck, 0 is ready to go.

Take a gentle breath in . . . and out.

Start tapping on the side of your hand. Repeat either in your mind or out loud.

Side of the Hand: Even though I feel stuck,
and part of me just doesn't want to do this,
I acknowledge myself and how I feel.

Even though I'm procrastinating,
and I feel a little guilty about it,
I choose to be kind to myself.

Even though I can't seem to find the motivation,
I'm open to finding my flow again.

Eyebrow: This lack of motivation
Side of the Eye: This feeling of being stuck
Under the Eye: I keep putting it off
Under the Nose: It feels too hard to start
Under the Mouth: All this resistance
Collarbone: It's easier to just avoid it
Under the Arm: This procrastination loop
Top of the Head: I feel so blocked

Eyebrow: What's behind this procrastination?
Side of the Eye: Maybe it's fear of making a mistake
Under the Eye: Things not going as planned
Under the Nose: Just not wanting to do it
Under the Mouth: I notice the pressure I put on myself . . .
Collarbone: and any remaining resistance

Under the Arm: Whatever comes up is ready to be cleared
Top of the Head: I'm finding a new way forward

Eyebrow: What if it's safe to start?
Side of the Eye: Even just a tiny first step
Under the Eye: Releasing the pressure to be perfect
Under the Nose: It doesn't have to be a certain way
Under the Mouth: I can just start
Collarbone: My nervous system can relax
Under the Arm: I'm open to this being easier than I think
Top of the Head: Allowing my energy to start to flow

Eyebrow: I'm letting go of this block
Side of the Eye: I can handle this
Under the Eye: My natural drive is returning
Under the Nose: It feels good to make progress
Under the Mouth: Even if it's one small step at a time
Collarbone: Feeling clear and ready
Under the Arm: I'm on my way
Top of the Head: Feeling motivated and capable now

Gently stop tapping and let your hands rest. Take a deep breath in . . . and let it out slowly.

Check back in with yourself. Where's that stuck feeling on the 0-to-10 scale now? Notice if the task feels even a little more approachable.

You've just unlocked the energy that was trapped in resistance.

For a guided audio version of this Tapping meditation, visit www.thetappingsolution.com/rewired.

To Remember . . .

The Core Insight: *Your lack of motivation is not a character flaw; it's a protection signal from your nervous system. Procrastination is often a "freeze" response triggered by underlying emotions like overwhelm or fear of failure. You don't need to find more willpower. Your power lies in your ability to clear the emotional static that is blocking your natural drive and energy.*

The Practice: *Stop trying to force yourself into action. Instead, ask the real question: "What emotional roadblock is getting in my way?" Is it overwhelm? Fear of not doing it perfectly? Resentment? Your practice is to tap on that* feeling *first. By clearing the emotional debris before you begin, you remove the internal friction, allowing your natural motivation to surface effortlessly.*

CHAPTER 11

When You Beat Yourself Up

Turning Self-Criticism into Self-Compassion

Imagine if you had a roommate who followed you around all day saying things like:

"Nice job on that presentation, except for the part where you said 'um' three times. Everyone definitely noticed."

"Oh, you're wearing that? Bold choice."

"Remember when you tried this before and failed? Just saying."

"Sarah did it better. And faster. With better hair."

You'd evict them immediately, right? Maybe even change the locks and get a restraining order.

Now, we all have this roommate. The one we'd never willingly choose.

They live in our heads rent-free, offering unsolicited commentary on everything we do, think, or attempt. At least a real bad roommate might occasionally wash a dish or take out the trash. But our inner critic? They just sit on the couch of our consciousness, eating chips and pointing out our flaws.

And somehow, we've not only accepted them as a permanent resident, but we've started believing they're telling us important truths.

This constant inner criticism is one of the most persistent Reactive Loops in the human experience, an automatic stress response that fires every time you attempt something new, make a mistake, or even dare to feel good about yourself.

The weird part is how normal this feels. We're so used to this constant commentary that we barely notice it anymore. It's like living next to train tracks: eventually, you stop hearing the trains.

But what if you could serve an eviction notice? What if that critical voice that's been squatting in your mental space could finally be shown the door?

The Overprotective Bodyguard Who Got Confused

Here's the plot twist about your inner critic: They think they're helping.

I know, I know. It doesn't feel helpful when they're listing your failures at 2 P.M. on a Tuesday when you're trying to finish up that work project or pick your kids up from school. But stick with me.

Our inner critic is like a bodyguard hired on the day of a crisis. Maybe they were hired after that scathing performance review from your boss when you were 30. Or after the heartbreak from your first love when you were 18. Or maybe they've been with you since the playground. The point is, a moment of pain put them on duty.

Back then, their job made sense:

- "If I criticize you first, no one else's criticism will hurt as much."
- "If I keep you small, you won't be a target."
- "If I remind you of past failures, you won't risk failing again."
- "If I point out your flaws, maybe you'll fix them before anyone notices."

It's protection through prevention. This is how Reactive Loops form—in moments of emotional intensity, your nervous system creates rapid-response patterns to prevent future pain. The amygdala essentially hardwires these protective responses, creating neural superhighways that bypass your rational mind.

But a bodyguard who keeps you safe by never letting you leave the house isn't a very fun companion, is it?

The problem is, the crisis is over. The dangers your inner critic is protecting you from—that old boss, that past relationship, that one public failure—they're all just memories, not active threats. But your bodyguard hasn't gotten the memo that things are different now.

They're still operating on a crisis protocol written in a moment of panic, applying outdated rules to your present-day life. Their job description was written in the frantic handwriting of a past emergency: *"Whatever it takes, never let that specific feeling happen again."*

This is why your inner critic gets loudest right before you do something brave.

Starting a business? → *"Remember when your lemonade stand failed?"*
Applying for a dream job? → *"You're not qualified and everyone will know."*
Falling in love? → *"Remember how that ended last time?"*

Your bodyguard thinks they're saving your life. But they're actually just preventing you from living a full life.

When do you think your bodyguard was hired? Can you trace it back to a specific time, event, or relationship in your life?

The Neuroscience of Self-Criticism

When self-criticism takes over, your body may feel tense, heavy, and restless, like you're bracing for failure even when nothing is wrong. In your mind, it feels like being trapped in a loop: replaying mistakes, doubting yourself, and struggling to believe any success counts.

Here's what's actually happening in your brain when self-criticism takes over:

- **The Default Mode Network Hijack:** Your Default Mode Network (DMN), the brain regions active during rest and self-reflection, becomes hyperactive during self-criticism. Instead of promoting healthy self-awareness, this hyperactivity creates a feedback loop that fuels rumination and reinforces negative self-beliefs.
- **The Anterior Cingulate Cortex Overload:** This brain region, your brain's "error detector" region, becomes hyper-alert—flagging even small missteps as big problems.
- **The Dopamine Depletion:** Chronic self-criticism blunts the brain's reward system, making dopamine signaling less effective. As a result, achievements feel flat instead of satisfying. It's like your brain stops registering your wins.
- **The Cortisol Cascade:** Self-critical rumination activates the stress response, releasing cortisol. Over time, elevated cortisol can weaken the hippocampus (involved in memory and self-concept), making it harder to build positive self-narratives.

THE INNER CRITIC PERSONALITY QUIZ

I want you to try a little experiment. Right now, say something genuinely nice about yourself out loud. Something you're proud of.

"I'm a really caring friend."

"I'm great at my job."

"I handled that situation well."

Did you hear it? That immediate "Yeah, but . . ." that followed? That's your inner critic, and it's faster than you think.

Now let's get acquainted with its favorite phrases, preferred topics, and signature moves. Check which of these sound familiar:

The Greatest Hits Collection:

- ❏ "You're not _____ enough" (smart/pretty/talented/qualified)
- ❏ "Who do you think you are?"
- ❏ "Remember what happened last time?"
- ❏ "Everyone can see you're faking it"
- ❏ "They're just being nice"
- ❏ "You always mess this up"
- ❏ "Why can't you be more like _____?"
- ❏ "This is why you can't have nice things"

Their Favorite Topics:

- ❏ Your appearance ("You look tired/old/wrong")
- ❏ Your intelligence ("That was a dumb thing to say")
- ❏ Your relationships ("They don't really like you")
- ❏ Your work ("Everyone knows you're incompetent")
- ❏ Your potential ("You'll never amount to anything")
- ❏ Your past ("Remember when you failed at . . .")
- ❏ Your worth ("You don't deserve good things")

Their Preferred Timing:

- ❑ Right before something important
- ❑ When you're trying to sleep
- ❑ After any minor mistake
- ❑ When someone compliments you
- ❑ When you're about to take a risk
- ❑ In the mirror
- ❑ All. The. Time.

Look at your checkmarks. That's your inner critic's personality profile. Every checkmark represents a Reactive Loop, a pattern so familiar your brain runs it on autopilot.

THE CURIOSITY CURE: HOW TO DISARM THE CRITIC

The most effective way to disarm the inner critic is to shift your stance from judgment to observation. This is a strategy I call the **Curiosity Cure**.

THE RULE:
Judgment stops the healing process; curiosity accelerates it.

When you hear that critical voice and judge it ("I shouldn't feel this way"; "This is so negative"), you activate more stress and lock the pattern in place. Curiosity, however, keeps your nervous system open and creates space for change.

What to Do: The next time your critic gets loud, replace your usual self-judgment with one simple phrase: **"Isn't that interesting . . ."**

For example: "Isn't that interesting? My mind is telling me I'm not qualified for this job." This simple shift takes you out of the battle and into the role of a compassionate scientist observing a pattern. From that curious, calmer state, you can begin to rewire it.

The Documentary That Almost Didn't Exist

Let me tell you about the moment I almost let *my* overprotective bodyguard win.

It was 2007, and I had this burning desire to create a documentary about Tapping. The vision was crystal clear; I could see how it would help people, how it would spread this incredible technique to those who needed it.

Have you ever had a big dream or idea that fired you up, only to quickly feel that spark dimmed by the doubts and insecurities that flooded your mind?

Every morning I'd wake up excited about the possibility, and within minutes, my inner critic would launch its protection protocol:

"You've never made a film." (True, but trying to keep me safe from embarrassment.)

"You don't have the resources." (Also true, and trying to save me from financial risk.)

"Real filmmakers know what they're doing." (Attempting to protect me from being seen as a fraud.)

"This is going to be embarrassing." (Classic bodyguard move—prevent all possible humiliation.)

Every day I woke up with this battle raging. The vision pulling me forward, my inner bodyguard pulling me back. "I'm trying to save you here!" it would insist. "Remember, we don't do things we're not already good at. That's the rule!"

I'd reached a Choice Point: that moment where I could either fall into my familiar Reactive Loop (listen to the critic, stay safe, stay small) or Interrupt the pattern and create a new Rewired Response.

And here's what saved me: I had a tool that could interrupt this pattern at the neurological level.

Why Tapping Silences the Critic (Without Firing Your Protector)

Here's what's actually happening in your brain when your inner critic gets loud:

Your amygdala (alarm center) perceives a threat—usually to your ego or identity. It signals your nervous system: "Danger! They might fail/be rejected/look foolish!" Your inner critic jumps in with its protection strategy: "I'll criticize them first! I'll keep them small! I'll remind them of past failures! That'll keep them safe!"

This all happens in milliseconds, below conscious awareness. By the time you notice the critical thoughts, your nervous system is already in protection mode.

Tapping works because it speaks directly to this system. When you tap while acknowledging the critical thoughts, several things happen simultaneously:

1. **The Biochemical Shift:** Tapping on acupoints sends calming signals through your nervous system, reducing cortisol by up to 43 percent. Your amygdala actually calms down.
2. **The Pattern Interrupt:** The physical sensation of Tapping disrupts the automatic Reactive Loop. It's like changing the channel on the criticism broadcast, physically disrupting the neural pathway mid-fire and creating what neuroscientists call a "window of reconsolidation."
3. **The Safety Signal:** The bilateral stimulation (tapping on both sides of the body) signals safety to your primitive brain. Your system gets the message: "We're okay. We can lower the shields."
4. **The Rewiring Opportunity:** With your nervous system calm and the pattern interrupted, you can install new Rewired Responses. Instead of "I'm not good enough," you can wire in "I'm learning and growing."

Every time I tapped on my documentary fears, I was rewiring my response to self-doubt. Not eliminating my inner protector (they were just trying to help), but updating their job description.

I ended up going for it. Did it go perfectly? No. I ended up maxing out credit cards. I fumbled through the process. I made rookie mistakes.

But that documentary? It went on to change millions of lives. It launched everything: our books, our app, this entire movement.

None of it would have happened if I'd let my inner critic do what it thought was best—keep me safe by keeping me small.

Name one specific opportunity or moment of joy that your inner critic has stolen from you. Allow yourself to feel the weight of that cost for just a moment–and let it fuel you to interrupt the pattern to find a new way forward.

The Facebook Post That Started a Revolution

Sometimes transformation looks dramatic. Other times, it looks like Myra, sitting at her computer, typing words that would inspire thousands.

She'd been doing our "You Are Enough" Tapping meditation every day for eight days. Each session, she was hitting the same Choice Point: believe the critic saying "not enough" or tap toward a new truth.

"Tapping on 'You Are Enough' has been the most amazing experience for me," she wrote. "I have tapped on this every day for the past eight days. Yesterday I tapped on 'You Are Enough,' and afterwards I rated 0 on the scale."

Zero. From a lifetime of "not enough" to zero emotional charge in eight days.

Here's the neuroscience behind this: She wasn't just changing her thoughts. Through repeated Tapping, she was rewiring her nervous system's response. The neural pathway that said "not enough" was being overwritten with new programming: "enough, exactly as I am."

"This morning I feel like a different person. The world looks brighter. I keep stopping and staring out of the window with such joy and gladness in my heart that tears trickle down my cheeks, and I just let them. I feel so blessed with the burden of not being enough being lifted completely—because I am enough!!!"

Her post went viral in our community. The comments poured in from people recognizing their own "not enough" programming, their own Familiarity Trap of self-criticism.

That single post inspired us to create our "You Are Enough" Challenge (a challenge that involves repeating this one meditation every day, for a few days, to allow enough time for a true pattern interrupt), which has now helped thousands discover what Myra discovered: You can rewire a lifetime of self-criticism in just a few days.

The People-Pleasing Connection

Here's a pattern we see constantly: The louder your inner critic, the more you feel the need for external validation.

When Peggy started tapping daily, she discovered this connection firsthand. As her inner critic quieted, something unexpected happened: She stopped needing everyone else's approval.

"I am losing my bad habit of being a people pleaser and door mat," she reported. "I no longer need toxic people and energy vampires in my life!"

This makes perfect neurological sense. When your inner critic constantly signals "not enough," your nervous system desperately seeks external evidence that you're okay. You'll do anything for approval because approval temporarily provides a feeling of safety, which temporarily quiets the critic.

But when you rewire that inner "not enough" program? As Peggy told us, "I now have the strength and courage to stand alone, clear out the wrong people, and make room for the right people in my life!"

What a beautiful, heartwarming, deeply transformative result.

You don't need others to tell you you're enough when you finally believe it yourself.

The Comparison Trap (And How I Almost Lost Myself in It)

Another common Inner Critic pattern involves the comparison trap, where you can't help but compare yourself to others who seem to have it all figured out.

Let me tell you about my own journey with this, because for years I was caught in my own comparison trap with someone I deeply admired.

I discovered personal development through Tony Robbins. Tony Robbins is one of those larger-than-life figures who has cultivated a movement around him of successful people (like Serena Williams, Hugh Jackman, and others), who turn to him for help and inspiration.

I was that guy who found his mom's Tony Robbins audio tapes and became obsessed. Discovering his work was like opening a door to a completely new way of seeing the world. In fact, he's the man who introduced me to the concept of Tapping in the first place.

For the first couple of years after getting into his work, I felt like I needed to do everything *exactly* the way he said to do it. His routines, his eating habits, all of it. I wanted to model myself after this clearly successful and inspirational person.

And look, it's great to model someone who you feel aligned with, who you can learn from. Having mentors and learning from the best—that's how we grow. But somewhere along the way, I started losing myself in trying to be a 2nd-rate (or 18th-rate if we're really being honest) version of Tony instead of a 1st-rate version of Nick.

In this day and age with social media and constant comparison opportunities, it's so easy to get lost in trying to be someone else. We get inspired by others, which is beautiful, but then we lose ourselves trying to replicate their exact path, their exact style, their exact success.

And here's what we forget: You have to be YOU. You have to find your own way.

The plot twist in my story came years later. After doing my own work, following my heart, focusing on what I thought was important (not trying to impress anyone or be anyone else), I ended up meeting Tony in the most unexpected way.

It was after Sandy Hook. I was serving my community, helping because it felt right to do so. I was being myself and following my heart's calling. And Tony came to help.

Not because I tried to reach out to him or get someone to introduce me or orchestrate some meeting. I met my idol when I wasn't trying to meet my idol. And that meeting just so happened to spark a beautiful partnership that led to all sorts of beautiful things.

Later, I found myself at Tony's house, discussing the ways we could serve together. And during our meeting, Tony was scribbling notes nonstop. Page after page of notes.

I looked around the room and realized: I didn't even have anything to write with. "I should be taking notes," my inner critic whispered. "Tony's taking notes. Everyone important/smart/successful takes notes."

But then it hit me: I'm not a note-taker. Never have been. That's just not how I process information best. Tony was doing his thing, and I was doing mine. Nobody was doing anything wrong.

That moment crystallized something profound for me: My inner critic had been trying to turn me into someone else for years. Every "you should be more like . . ." thought was taking me further from my authentic self.

The beautiful full-circle moment? Tony ended up becoming the only outside investor in The Tapping Solution App. This partnership happened not because I successfully imitated him, but because I followed my own path, which led to creating something unique that he wanted to support.

Every time you compare yourself to others and try to be more like someone else, it is your inner critic saying, "See? They're doing it right. You're doing it wrong. You should be more like them." Your brain just thinks it is trying to help, because it experiences social comparison as an actual threat to your survival.

But here's the truth I learned: The magic happens when you stop trying to be a second-rate version of someone else and start being a first-rate version of yourself.

This comparison trap is part of the Great Forgetting—that collective amnesia where we've forgotten that our uniqueness is our power, not our problem. We've forgotten that the world needs first-rate versions of ourselves, not second-rate copies of others.

When you tap on these comparison traps, something shifts. You stop seeing other people's success as evidence of your failure. You start recognizing that their path is information, not instruction. You can be inspired without being imitative.

You learn that you can be yourself, in all the beauty that YOU are.

YOUR VERSION OF "TAKING NOTES"

What's your version of thinking you should be taking notes when that's not who you are?

Maybe you think you should:

- Be more outgoing like your successful colleague
- Have it all together like that Instagram mom
- Be as calm as your yoga teacher friend
- Build your business just like that entrepreneur you follow
- Travel the world like your cousin who seems to always be on another life-changing adventure

Now, go one step further. Who would you be, and what would you create, if you fully gave yourself permission to stop imitating and start being YOU? What is one thing you would do differently this week if you weren't trying to live up to someone else's highlight reel?

The Committee Gets New Management

Remember that critical roommate from the beginning of the chapter? Here's what nobody tells you: You can't actually evict them. They have a lifetime lease. They're part of the building.

But you can change the way they show up in your life. You can change their job description.

Instead of Chief Critic, they can become Thoughtful Advisor. Instead of Dream Crusher, they can be Risk Assessor. Instead of Constant Commentator, they can be Occasional Consultant.

The voice that says, "You can't do this" can become "What do you need to learn to do this?"

The voice that says, "Remember when you failed" can become "What did you learn from that experience?"

The voice that says, "You're not enough" can become "What support do you need to feel empowered?"

This isn't about positive thinking or affirmations that feel fake. It's about updating old programming that no longer serves you. It's about recognizing that the bodyguard you hired at age five needs a new job description for the now strong and capable adult version of yourself.

Your Inner Critic Rehabilitation Program

Ready to transform your inner critic from harsh prosecutor to helpful advisor? Here's your road map:

Phase 1: Recognition For the next 24 hours, just notice your critic. When do they speak up? What triggers them? What are their favorite phrases? No judgment—just observation.

Phase 2: Appreciation This sounds crazy, but thank your critic. "Thanks for trying to protect me." They've been working 24/7 for years trying to keep you safe. Misguided? Yes. Dedicated? Absolutely.

Phase 3: The Tapping Update When your critic gets loud, tap. Not to silence them, but to calm your nervous system while you update their programming:

"Even though my inner critic is saying [specific criticism], and I know they're trying to protect me, I'm safe in this moment to try a new way forward."

"Even though this part of me believes keeping me small keeps me safe, I appreciate their dedication, and I'm open to growing in new ways."

Phase 4: The New Job Description After tapping, give your critic a new role. Instead of preventing all risk, maybe they can help you assess reasonable risks. Instead of listing why you'll fail, maybe they can help you prepare. Same voice, new purpose.

If your inner critic got promoted to "Thoughtful Advisor," what would their first piece of valuable advice be?

Why You Don't Need to Actually Believe It (Yet)

Here's what nobody tells you: You don't have to believe the new programming at first. You just have to create space for it.

When I was tapping about my documentary fears, I didn't suddenly believe I was Spielberg. I just created enough calm in my nervous system to ask, "What if I could figure this out?"

When Myra started tapping on "You Are Enough," her critic argued back for days. But she kept creating that neurological space where a new truth could take root, and eventually the narrative shifted completely.

This is the power of the REWIRED process:

- **Recognize** the critical voice as an old Reactive Loop
- **Interrupt** the narrative with Tapping
- **Rewire** by installing new, more empowering beliefs

Every tap is a vote for the new programming. Every session makes the new neural pathway stronger. Every day makes the old critical voice quieter.

The Truth Hidden in Plain Sight

Here's what took me 20 years to fully understand: Your inner critic is evidence of how much you matter.

Think about it. This part of you has been working 24/7 for decades trying to keep you safe. Misguided? Yes. Outdated? Absolutely. But dedicated? Completely.

You have a part of you that cares so much about your well-being that it never takes a day off. It's been trying to protect you with the only tools it knows: criticism, comparison, and caution.

What happens when you give it better tools?

Myra found out. In eight days, her protector learned that "You are enough" was a better safety strategy than "You're not enough."

Peggy discovered it. Her inner critic learned that boundaries create more safety than people pleasing.

I experienced it. My protector learned that growth could be safe, that failure could be survivable, that dreams could be worth the risk.

Your Invitation to Self-Compassion

So here you are, reading about people who've transformed their inner critics and wondering if it's possible for you.

I can feel your critic trying to speak up from here, can't you?

Right on cue. Maybe it's: "This works for other people, but not for you" or "Your patterns are too deep" or "You've tried before and failed."

This is a Familiarity Trap in action. Your nervous system is running its favorite protection program. Your bodyguard is doing what they've always done. Trying to protect you from the disappointment of hoping.

But you're at a Choice Point right now. You can close this book and let your critic keep running your life. Or you can try something different.

What if that voice is wrong? Not bad, not evil, just . . . wrong? Operating on outdated information? Using old strategies that no longer serve you?

What if "You are enough" isn't a feel-good affirmation but a simple fact your protector hasn't learned yet?

What if your inner critic is ready for a new job; they just need someone to write the new job description?

What if that someone is you?

The documentary I almost didn't make has helped millions of people. But it never would have existed if I hadn't been willing to tap through the voice that was trying to keep me safe by keeping me small.

Your dreams, the ones your critic talks you out of, they matter too. The world needs what you have to offer. We need the version of you that emerges when your harsh inner critic becomes your compassionate inner advisor.

So keep tapping. Keep making that shift, one neural pathway at a time.

Until one day, like Myra, you look out your window and the way you see the whole world has changed.

Because the way you see yourself has.

Ready to see yourself in a whole new light?

Let's tap.

RECLAIMING *Your* FREEDOMS

The pattern we explored in this chapter doesn't just cause discomfort; it actively steals some of your 7 Freedoms. By using Tapping to rewire this pattern, you're not just getting rid of a problem—you're reclaiming your birthright to a full, vibrant life.

Take a moment to reflect: Which of these freedoms would open up the most for you if this pattern no longer had a hold on you?

- The freedom to experience emotions without being overwhelmed.
- The freedom to respond with wisdom instead of reacting from old wounds.
- The freedom to feel calm in situations that used to throw you.
- The freedom to access energy you didn't know you had.
- The freedom to feel at home and peaceful in your body.
- The freedom to trust yourself to handle whatever comes your way.
- The freedom to show up as your real self, not who you've been conditioned to be.

What is the first thing you would do, create, or experience with this newfound freedom?

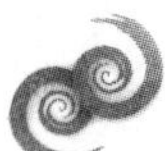

TAPPING SCRIPT: *From Self-Criticism to Self-Compassion*

Let's check in with that inner voice.

On a scale of 0 to 10, how loud or active is your inner critic right now? A 10 is "I believe everything it says" and 0 is "I notice it but it doesn't have power over me."

Take a gentle breath in . . . and out.

Start tapping on the side of your hand. Repeat either in your mind or out loud.

Side of the Hand: Even though a part of me is critical of myself,
and I feel like I'm not good enough,
I acknowledge all parts of me.

Even though this critical voice is so persistent,
I'm open to a new, more compassionate way.

Even though I'm so used to beating myself up,
and I'm nervous about what will happen if I stop,
I'm willing to explore new possibilities.

Eyebrow: This inner critic
Side of the Eye: This voice of self-doubt
Under the Eye: It always seems to be there
Under the Nose: It's so exhausting
Under the Mouth: I'm tired of getting in my own way . . .
Collarbone: and feeling like I'm not enough
Under the Arm: I simply notice this pattern
Top of the Head: It's an outdated protective mechanism

Eyebrow: Maybe in the past it did protect me . . .
Side of the Eye: but it's now keeping me small
Under the Eye: I am older and wiser now
Under the Nose: I can notice that critical voice . . .
Under the Mouth: but I don't have to believe everything I think
Collarbone: It's safe to step into my power
Under the Arm: I don't need more criticism . . .
Top of the Head: in order to move forward

Eyebrow: I choose self-compassion and courage instead
Side of the Eye: I am making room for my inner wisdom . . .
Under the Eye: which knows that I am enough . . .
Under the Nose: even in moments when I don't fully believe it
Under the Mouth: I release any excess pressure I put on myself
Collarbone: It is safe to grow
Under the Arm: It is safe to learn as I go
Top of the Head: It is safe to expand

Eyebrow: I choose to be kind to myself
Side of the Eye: I acknowledge how far I've already come
Under the Eye: I give myself the credit I deserve
Under the Nose: I am worthy and capable
Under the Mouth: I'm excited to see what I can do . . .
Collarbone: when I give myself the freedom to try
Under the Arm: I'm becoming a better friend to myself
Top of the Head: Feeling grounded and ready

Gently stop tapping and let your hands rest. Take a deep breath in . . . and let it out slowly.

Check in with that inner voice now. How strong is it now on the 0-to-10 scale?

You haven't silenced your protector; you've just started a new, more collaborative relationship.

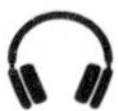 **For a guided audio version of this Tapping meditation, visit www.thetappingsolution.com/rewired.**

To Remember . . .

The Core Insight: *The hopeful truth is that your inner critic is not your enemy; it's an overprotective bodyguard running on outdated programming from the past. You don't have to defeat it. You have the power to calm your nervous system and give your protector a new, more supportive job description.*

The Practice: *When you hear that critical voice inside, treat it with curiosity, not judgment. Thank it for trying to keep you safe. Then, use Tapping on the feeling of "not being enough" or the self-doubt or the specific criticism you hear. This calms the underlying threat response, reminds your system that you are safe as you are, and creates the space to update your protector's role from "harsh critic" to "compassionate advisor."*

CHAPTER 12

When You're Just SO Tired

Restoring Energy at Its Source

"How are you?"

"Tired."

"But how *are* you?"

"I just told you. Tired."

Welcome to the modern exhaustion epidemic, where being tired isn't a temporary state; it's a personality trait.

This isn't the normal tired after an extra-long day. This isn't the understandable fatigue of new parents or shift workers. This is the kind of exhaustion where it seeps into every aspect of your life: the bone-deep, soul-level tired that sleep doesn't fix and coffee can't touch.

You've tried everything:

- Going to bed earlier (hello, 3 A.M. wake up!)
- Cutting back on activities (now you're tired *and* bored)
- More vitamins (your pee is very expensive now)
- Exercise for energy (with what energy exactly?)
- Positive thinking (toxic positivity is exhausting too)

Yet there you are, googling "why am I so tired all the time" at 2 A.M., using energy you don't have during daylight to search for energy you can't find.

This exhaustion isn't just a feeling; it's a Reactive Loop that's become so familiar, so constant, that you've forgotten what real energy feels like. You're living in the ultimate Familiarity Trap where being tired has become your identity.

We've normalized this persistent lack of energy to the point where when someone bounces into work genuinely energized, we assume they're faking it, taking something, or haven't been adulting long enough to know better.

But here's a fun fact that nobody mentions: Being exhausted all the time isn't normal. I know, shocking.

THE ENERGY AUDIT

Let's identify how low energy is showing up in your life. Check off which patterns feel true for you.

Physical Patterns:

- ❑ Heavy feeling in chest/shoulders
- ❑ Brain fog that coffee can't clear
- ❑ The 3 P.M. crash that feels like hitting a wall
- ❑ Waking up tired no matter how much you sleep
- ❑ Feeling like you're moving through mud
- ❑ "How are you?" "Tired." is your standard exchange

Mental Patterns:

- ❑ Everything feels like too much effort
- ❑ Simple decisions are exhausting
- ❑ Can't remember why anything matters
- ❑ Bedtime and wake time blur because you're tired all 24 hours
- ❑ Fantasizing about disappearing to a cabin in the woods
- ❑ Feeling like a phone on 2 percent battery all day

Emotional Patterns:

- ❑ Too tired to feel anything deeply
- ❑ Irritability is your default setting
- ❑ Zero enthusiasm for things you used to enjoy
- ❑ Canceling plans because showering felt like too much
- ❑ Feeling like you're letting everyone down by being tired
- ❑ Guilt about being tired making you more tired

Look at the items you just checked off. This isn't just a list; it's a map of how exhaustion is stealing from your life. Pick one physical, mental, or emotional pattern that feels most true for you right now. Get specific: What is the real, tangible cost of this pattern? Is it the joy of a hobby you no longer have energy for? Is it your patience with your children? Is it your confidence at work?

When Your Power Grid Is Down

Here's the truth bomb that changed everything: Your exhaustion isn't because you're doing too much. It's because your cellular power plants are actually operating at half capacity.

Excuse me while I get nerdy for a moment. But understanding this changes everything.

Scientists discovered that when your nervous system detects stress, your mitochondria—the actual power generators in your cells—can cut energy production by up to 50 percent. In minutes.

But when the stress signals are removed? Energy production rebounds just as quickly.

And that is huge.

When your nervous system is in chronic stress mode, your mitochondria (those tiny power plants in your cells) literally produce less energy.

Here's the mechanism: Stress triggers your hypothalamic-pituitary-adrenal (HPA) axis, flooding your system with cortisol. This chronic stress signal forces your mitochondria to switch from energy production to cellular defense, rationing the fuel available for your daily life. All your resources divert to survival.

Let that sink in. Your actual cellular power plants are operating at reduced capacity because your nervous system thinks you're being chased by bears all day.

Every worry, every stress, every "what if" is dimming your power.

Like someone's going through your house flipping off light switches:

Worried about money? Click—there goes 10 percent of your energy.

Conflict with your partner? Click—another 15 percent offline.

Perfectionism running in the background? Click—20 percent more gone.

No wonder you're tired. You're trying to run your whole life on the power equivalent of a nightlight.

Your nervous system is convinced that e-mails are emergencies, that traffic is a threat, that your to-do list is actively trying to take you down.

Your cellular power plants are screaming: "We can't sustain this! We're rationing energy! Nonessential functions are being shut down!"

Nonessential functions like . . . feeling alive. Having enthusiasm. Remembering why you wanted to do any of this in the first place.

Your body has gotten so used to operating in emergency mode that exhaustion feels normal.

This is the **Great Forgetting** in action. We've forgotten what it feels like to have real energy. We've forgotten that vitality is our birthright, not a luxury reserved for the young or the privileged. We've accepted this cellular-level exhaustion as "just how adults feel," when it's actually our nervous systems stuck in perpetual crisis mode.

And so every morning presents a Choice Point: Accept the fatigue as "just how you are" or interrupt the pattern that's draining your cellular batteries.

THE LIES TIRED PEOPLE TELL

- "I just need a good night's sleep." (It's not about sleep.)
- "I'll rest this weekend." (You won't.)
- "It's just a busy season." (It's been five years.)
- "Everyone's tired." (Not like this they're not.)
- "I'm just getting older." (Exhaustion isn't normal aging.)

Which one do you tell yourself the most?

The Woman Who Found Her Second Wind at 6 P.M.

Eva dragged herself through the front door after work, feeling that ready-for-bed-at-6-P.M. kind of exhaustion where taking off your shoes feels like too much effort, so you just sit on the couch fully dressed, staring at nothing.

But instead of surrendering to the couch coma, Eva tried something that seemed almost insultingly simple. She pulled up an "Instant Boost of Energy" Tapping session on her phone.

Minutes later (not hours, not after a nap, not after mainlining espresso), she felt like she'd actually had that nap.

"I feel like I've had a nap! Truly amazing feeling," she told us.

No caffeine crash. No jittery aftermath. No lying in bed later, exhausted but wired. Just . . . energy. Real, sustainable, "I can actually enjoy my evening" energy.

If you could have an "instant boost of energy" right now, what is the one thing you would do with it?

The Plot Twist

Here's what fascinates me about every exhaustion story we receive: The energy was there all along. It never left. It had just been diverted, suppressed, or short-circuited by stress responses that the nervous system thought would keep you safe.

This explains something that makes no sense otherwise: How can someone tap on their face for five minutes and suddenly feel energized?

They're not creating fake energy or fooling themselves. They're working with their nervous system to turn their cellular power plants back on.

That night at 6 P.M., Eva didn't create new energy from thin air. She removed the blocks that were suppressing her existing energy.

It's kind of like having a kinked garden hose. You don't need more water pressure, you just need to unkink the hose. Tapping unkinks your energy flow by calming the stress signals that are constraining it.

Your exhaustion might not be about needing more sleep or better vitamins. It might be about stress signals that are telling your cells to run on power-saver mode.

This illustrates a key principle from our REWIRED framework: You don't need to generate new energy through force. You need to Recognize the stress-driven Reactive Loops draining your power, Interrupt them with Tapping, and Rewire your system back to its natural energy-abundant state.

THE PARKING BRAKE PRINCIPLE

This cellular energy drain is a hidden cost to our vitality, one that explains why we're so exhausted even when we haven't "done" that much. I call it the **Parking Brake Principle**.

THE RULE:
You aren't tired because you're doing too much; you're tired because you're doing everything with the brakes on.

Operating in survival mode applies constant internal friction–anxiety, worry, muscle tension–to every single action. It's like driving your car with the parking brake engaged. You have to floor the gas pedal just to move, burning massive amounts of fuel and wearing down the engine. This is why you feel so drained at the end of the day.

The solution isn't to do less. It's to use Tapping to release the brake. When you clear the underlying stress, you reclaim all the energy that was being wasted on internal friction.

The Hidden Energy Vampires

We need to talk about what's really draining you, because it's not always what you think.

Sure, your schedule is full. Yes, the kids are exhausting. Of course work is demanding. But that's not necessarily the whole picture of why you're tired.

You're tired because your nervous system is working overtime on invisible threats you probably aren't even aware of.

Here are a few examples of hidden energy vampires that could be affecting your life. Read through the list and notice which ones resonate with you, which make you say, "Oooh, that's me!"

- **The Perfectionism Drain:** Every task requires 150 percent effort because 100 percent might not be enough. Your mitochondria are working overtime for a boss (you) who's never satisfied.
- **The Hypervigilance Hemorrhage:** Constantly scanning for what might go wrong, what you might have forgotten, who might be upset with you. It's exhausting being your own security detail.

- **The Emotional Labor Leak:** Managing everyone else's feelings while suppressing your own. You're running an emotional air traffic control center 24/7.
- **The Comparison Vampire:** Checking social media and finding 17 new ways you're failing at life. Each comparison drains a little more life force.
- **The Resentment Reactor:** That low-grade anger at a situation that you can't quite resolve. It's like driving with the parking brake on—you're burning extra fuel just to move forward.

Each of these runs constantly in the background, like apps draining your phone battery. You might not even notice them anymore, but your mitochondria sure do.

Take a moment to slow down and reflect (or even jot down a few notes to reflect on further later):

Which vampires from the list are draining your battery? Which are most present in your life? What would it be like to go through one day without the "Perfectionist Drain" or the "Resentment Reactor" running in the background?

The 65-Year Energy Revolution

Before you read about 65-year-old Linda's transformation, let me ask you something:

How long have you been tired? When did it start? Can you even remember? Or has exhaustion become so familiar that you've forgotten what energy feels like?

When did "tired" become your identity instead of your temporary state?

Well, Linda's story destroys every excuse about being "too old" or "too tired" or "too *anything*" to change.

At 65, after decades of "less-than, never-good-enough issues," she started Tapping. Not with grand expectations. Not with a complex protocol.

Here's what she reported to us after just simple, consistent Tapping before bed: "My energy is amazing, as are feelings of positivity and well-being. I'm feeling so *CAPABLE* now."

At 65, after a lifetime of energy-draining self-criticism, she's not just less tired. She's "*amazing.*" She's "CAPABLE." She's discovering energy reserves from within she didn't know existed.

In Linda's own words: "Tapping releases up so much heavy, draining energy."

That's the secret. That's what this really is all about.

You're not exactly creating energy. You're *releasing* what's been blocking it from flowing through you. All those years of self-doubt, criticism, and not-enough-ness? They weren't just emotional burdens for Linda. They were cellular energy drains.

And when they were cleared? Her energy returned. Along with it, her feelings of positivity returned, her quality of life returned, her sense of empowerment returned.

Your Cellular Power Plant Revival

When you tap while acknowledging exhaustion, here's what happens at the cellular level:

1. **Stress Signals Reduce:** Cortisol drops, telling your mitochondria the crisis is over.
2. **Energy Production Normalizes:** Your cellular power plants shift from emergency mode to sustainable energy production.
3. **Inflammation Decreases:** Chronic inflammation (an energy vampire) starts to resolve.
4. **Cellular Repair Activates:** Energy previously diverted to stress responses becomes available for healing and restoration.
5. **Natural Rhythms Return:** Your body remembers its natural energy cycles instead of the flatlined exhaustion you've been experiencing.

This isn't temporary energy like caffeine. This is your body remembering how to generate sustainable power.

The Permission You've Been Waiting For

Before we tap, I need to give you permission for something:

You're allowed to be tired.

I know that seems to contradict everything I've just said, but stick with me. Part of why you're so exhausted is that you're exhausted by being exhausted. You're spending energy feeling guilty about having no energy.

You're fighting your tiredness, judging it, trying to power through it. That's like trying to put out a fire with gasoline.

So here's your permission slip: You're allowed to be exactly as tired as you are. You don't have to pretend. You don't have to fake energy. You don't have to be the person who has it all together.

You can be tired. And from that place of acceptance and self-compassion, paradoxically, real energy can start to flow again.

The Energy You Didn't Know You Had

Here's my promise to you:

Underneath your exhaustion—beneath the brain fog, beyond the 3 P.M. crash, behind the "I just can't" feeling—your natural energy is waiting for you.

Not the fake, jittery energy of your fourth espresso. Not the forced enthusiasm of pretending everything's fine. But real, sustainable, "I actually want to do things and live my life" kind of energy.

Eva found it in minutes. Linda uncovered it at age 65.

They didn't create this energy. They removed what was blocking it. They unkinked the hose. They told their mitochondria: "You can go back to normal operations now."

Every one of them hit the same Choice Point you're facing now: Accept exhaustion as permanent *or* interrupt the pattern that's maintaining it.

They chose to interrupt. They chose to tap. They chose to discover who they are when they're not running on empty.

RECLAIMING *Your* FREEDOMS

The pattern we explored in this chapter doesn't just cause discomfort; it actively steals some of your 7 Freedoms. By using Tapping to rewire this pattern, you're not just getting rid of a problem–you're reclaiming your birthright to a full, vibrant life.

Take a moment to reflect: Which of these freedoms would open up the most for you if this pattern no longer had a hold on you?

- The freedom to experience emotions without being overwhelmed.
- The freedom to respond with wisdom instead of reacting from old wounds.
- The freedom to feel calm in situations that used to throw you.
- The freedom to access energy you didn't know you had.
- The freedom to feel at home and peaceful in your body.
- The freedom to trust yourself to handle whatever comes your way.
- The freedom to show up as your real self, not who you've been conditioned to be.

What is the first thing you would do, create, or experience with this newfound freedom?

The Spontaneous Joy Circuit

Sometimes when you restore power, you don't just get functionality—you get fireworks.

Karrie was having a typical afternoon energy crash when she decided to tap instead of reaching for coffee. Halfway through the session, something unexpected happened:

"I felt this huge burst of excitement and spontaneously burst into laughter. I was literally just laughing from sheer joy and excitement."

This wasn't forced positivity. This was what happens when you suddenly have energy to spare—joy becomes possible again. Play becomes possible. Spontaneous laughter on a Tuesday afternoon becomes possible.

"That has only happened to me once before during a hot yoga class!" she added.

When your power grid is fully functional, you don't just survive—you light up.

Karrie's story reminds us that getting your energy back isn't just about being able to do your laundry or answer e-mails. It's about reopening the circuits for joy, spontaneity, and laughter.

What is a "spontaneous joy" you feel you've lost to exhaustion? Is it singing loudly in the car? Dancing in the kitchen while making dinner? Getting lost in a creative project for hours? What would it feel like to welcome that playful part of yourself back home?

The Choice in This Moment

It's 3:17 P.M. as I write this. Prime exhaustion time. The time when most of us either push through with willpower or surrender to the slump.

So here you are, probably reading this through tired eyes, maybe on your third cup of coffee, possibly fantasizing about a nap you know won't help.

Your inner skeptic (who's also tired) is saying: "This won't work. You're different. Your exhaustion is real."

And you know what? Your exhaustion *is* real. It's biologically, cellularly, mitochondrially real.

But so is your capacity to shift it.

The choice is yours. You can close this book, drag yourself to the kitchen for coffee number who knows, and keep wondering why everyone else seems to have more energy than you. Or you can take a few minutes right now, tired as you are, and start flipping those circuit breakers back on.

Because right now, this exhausted, tired version of you? You're not really living. You're existing. You're missing your life because you don't have the energy to participate in it. Your kids, your dreams, your potential, they all need the version of you that isn't running on 2 percent battery.

And your cellular power plants are ready to come back online. Your natural rhythms are waiting to return. Your energy—your real, sustainable, makes-life-worth-living energy—is right there, just beneath the stress signals that have been suppressing it.

So, here is your Choice Point. You can accept the 3 P.M. slump as your destiny. Or you can take the next three minutes and send a direct memo to your mitochondria: *The crisis is over. It's time to turn the power back on.*

Ready to flip the switch?

Let's tap.

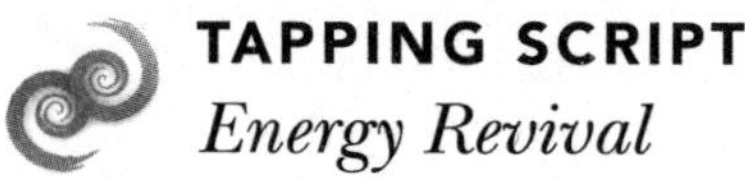

TAPPING SCRIPT: *Energy Revival*

Let's check in with your energy levels.

On a scale of 0 to 10, where 10 is "completely and utterly exhausted" and 0 is "energized," how do you feel right now?

Take a gentle breath in . . . and out.

Start tapping on the side of your hand. Repeat either in your mind or out loud.

Side of the Hand: Even though I feel so deeply tired,
I acknowledge my body and how I feel.

Even though I'm so tired of being tired,
and I've been running on empty for so long,
I choose to be gentle and patient with myself.

Even though I feel stuck in this exhaustion,
I am open to turning my power back on.

Eyebrow: This exhaustion
Side of the Eye: Like my battery is low
Under the Eye: A lack of energy
Under the Nose: There are a lot of things that drain me
Under the Mouth: My energy goes in so many directions
Collarbone: When life feels like too much . . .
Under the Arm: it's easy to lose myself
Top of the Head: I acknowledge this pattern

Eyebrow: I start to notice what's stealing my energy
Side of the Eye: Maybe it's trying to solve everyone's problems
Under the Eye: Maybe it's perfectionism
Under the Nose: Maybe the world just feels heavy
Under the Mouth: I've been holding on to so much . . .
Collarbone: and it's only holding me down
Under the Arm: I'm ready to begin to let go . . .
Top of the Head: and come back to my power

Eyebrow: Where my focus goes...
Side of the Eye: my energy flows
Under the Eye: I notice what I can control . . .
Under the Nose: and choose to take action
Under the Mouth: I notice what I can't control . . .
Collarbone: and begin to let go and let be
Under the Arm: It's safe to release these patterns
Top of the Head: It's safe to reclaim my power

Eyebrow: As I relax my body . . .
Side of the Eye: and feel this sense of safety . . .
Under the Eye: my energy starts to build
Under the Nose: I have the energy I need . . .
Under the Mouth: for life to feel brighter again
Collarbone: I open up to new possibilities . . .
Under the Arm: and spontaneous moments of joy
Top of the Head: It's safe to live more fully

Gently stop tapping and let your hands rest. Take a deep breath in . . . and let it out slowly.

Check back in with your body. Where is your energy level on the 0-to-10 scale now? Notice any small shifts—a little less fogginess, a little more lightness. If you feel better, your new number will be lower.

You've just reminded your body how to generate its own sustainable power.

 **For a guided audio version of this Tapping meditation, visit www.thetappingsolution.com/rewired.**

To Remember

The Core Insight: *Exhaustion isn't just about a lack of sleep; it's often a sign that your nervous system is stuck in survival mode, forcing your cellular power plants to operate at reduced capacity. The hopeful truth is that your energy isn't gone; it's just been suppressed by stress. You have the ability to turn the power back on and feel the energy flow again.*

The Practice: *Stop trying to "power through" fatigue. Instead, see your exhaustion as a signal from your body that it needs a nervous system reset. Your practice is to use Tapping to address the underlying stress and release the hidden drains on your system. Tapping sends a direct message to your cells that the emergency is over, allowing your natural energy to flow again.*

CHAPTER 13

When Sleep Refuses to Come

Reclaiming Deep, Restorative Rest

There's a special kind of loneliness that happens at 3:17 A.M.

You know the exact time because you've been watching those red digits mock you for the past hour and 43 minutes. The rest of the world is unconscious, lost in dreams you can't access. Even your anxious friend who's always up late finally posted her last Instagram story two hours ago.

It's just you, the darkness, and that infuriating awareness that every minute you're awake is another minute less before your alarm goes off.

You've already done the math. If you fall asleep *right now*, you'll get 3 hours and 24 minutes. Not great, but survivable.

3:18 A.M. Make that 3 hours and 23 minutes.

This is your nightly Reactive Loop in action: Check time. Calculate remaining sleep. Panic about lack of sleep. Become more awake from panic. Check time again.

Meanwhile, your brain has decided this is the perfect time to run through its Greatest Hits Collection:

- That embarrassing thing you said in 2011
- Everything that could go wrong tomorrow

- A sudden, urgent need to reorganize your entire life
- Deep philosophical questions about existence
- Whether you remembered to lock the door (you did, you've checked three times)

You're exhausted. Your body is begging for sleep. But your mind? Your mind is throwing a party, and everyone's invited except unconsciousness.

Every single night, you hit the same Choice Point: Do you fall into the familiar pattern of fighting for sleep? Or do you try something radically different?

The Cruel Mathematics of Insomnia

Here's what makes sleeplessness particularly sadistic: The harder you try to sleep, the more awake you become.

It's like quicksand. The more you struggle, the deeper you sink into wakefulness. Every desperate attempt to force sleep—counting, breathing, visualizing peaceful scenes—just adds another layer of alertness.

This is the ultimate Familiarity Trap. Your brain knows this dance: Try to sleep → Fail → Try harder → Fail worse. It's exhausting and ineffective, but it's what you've always done. And to your nervous system, familiar equals safe. Even when it's keeping you miserably awake. The mere act of lying down triggers your sympathetic nervous system, releasing norepinephrine and cortisol—the exact opposite of what you need for sleep.

Jane understood this special torture. She could see from her fitness tracker that her sleep was a mess. The data didn't lie: restless nights, minimal deep sleep, the kind of numbers that explain why you feel like you're moving through molasses all day.

But after just three nights of Tapping for sleep, everything changed.

"Oh my goodness. The difference to my energy after the three days sleep Tapping. I can see from my fitness tracker my sleep is improved."

Jane hit her Choice Point and chose differently. Instead of another night of sheep-counting futility, she chose to Interrupt the pattern with Tapping. And her nervous system responded by Rewiring its entire approach to sleep.

The real test came when she had to wake up at 5:45 A.M. for work—usually a recipe for a terrible night of anxious pre-alarm insomnia.

"Normally that would mean a poor night's sleep and difficulty getting up," she told us. "Not today. Slept soundly until my alarm, did the Instant Boost of Happiness Tapping meditation, and I feel amazing."

From data-documented poor sleep to "I feel amazing" in three nights.

That's the REWIRED process in action: Recognize the sleepless night pattern, Interrupt with Tapping, Rewire toward restful sleep.

THE INSOMNIAC'S REALITY CHECK

Quick quiz: How many of these are part of your nightly routine?

- ❑ Calculating remaining sleep time every 10 minutes
- ❑ Mentally writing tomorrow's to-do list at 2 A.M.
- ❑ Staring at the ceiling until you've memorized every pattern there is to find
- ❑ Googling "why can't I sleep" on your phone
- ❑ Getting irrationally angry at your partner's peaceful breathing
- ❑ Considering just getting up because "what's the point"
- ❑ Promising yourself you'll go to bed earlier tomorrow

When Counting Sheep Becomes an Olympic Sport

John drives trucks loaded with explosives for a living.

Let that sink in for a moment. When John doesn't sleep well, it's not just about feeling groggy at his desk job. It's about staying alert while hauling cargo that could level a city block.

After major surgery, his sleep disappeared. Not the gentle "I wake up once or twice" kind of insomnia. The dangerous "I'm operating heavy machinery on no sleep" kind.

"I was falling asleep behind the wheel," he shared with us. "When a wreck with that kind of cargo happens, it never turns out good."

John knew it was serious. The stakes were high. He recognized this pattern wasn't sustainable. At his Choice Point—to risk his life and others' or to try something new—he chose to Interrupt the pattern. And so, he started Tapping.

"It worked the first time I used it and has continued to work without fail every night."

Here's my favorite part of the story John shared with us. Usually, John makes it through all of the Tapping before going to sleep. But then . . . "One night my wife came to bed and said I was laying on my back with my fingertips on my collarbone, and I was just sawing logs."

He'd fallen asleep mid-Tapping session. Literally mid-tap. His body had gotten so used to the sleep signal that Tapping created, he couldn't even finish the meditation before unconsciousness claimed him.

If this isn't a sign of a nervous system being completely Rewired, I don't know what is. The new pattern was so strong that just starting to tap triggered sleep automatically.

John knew he couldn't keep operating trucks on no sleep.

But what about you? What are you operating on no sleep? Your life? Your relationships? Your kids? Your career?

When did "running on fumes" become your normal operating system?

Your Brain's Night Shift Security Guard

Let me paint you a picture of what's actually happening during those wide-awake nights:

Your conscious mind wants to sleep. It's exhausted, rational, knows that rest is essential. This is the part of you doing the sheep counting, trying the breathing exercises, thinking, "I really need to sleep."

But your subconscious has hired a security guard—let's call him Steve—whose job is to keep you safe. And Steve? Steve works the night shift with the dedication of someone who's had *way* too much coffee.

Steve's logic goes like this:

- "Unconsciousness means vulnerability."
- "We can't protect ourselves if we're asleep."
- "What if something important happens?"
- "What if we miss a threat?"
- "Better safe than sleeping."

This hypervigilance is your nervous system stuck in a Reactive Loop that probably made sense once, maybe during a stressful period when you needed to stay alert. But now it's become your Familiarity Trap, running every single night whether there's actual danger or not.

Steve means well. He's trying to protect you. But Steve is operating on survival software written for a world where letting your guard down at night meant becoming something's midnight snack.

This is your Familiarity Trap personified. Steve's been doing this job so long, he can't imagine any other way. To him, hypervigilance equals safety. Sleep equals danger. It's familiar, therefore it must be best.

This is a prime example of the Great Forgetting. We've forgotten that sleep is supposed to be natural, automatic, effortless. Our ancestors didn't need sleep apps or white noise machines. They laid down when tired and woke when rested. But we've forgotten this basic biological function, turning it into another thing we can "fail" at.

The problem? You're not in a cave anymore. The biggest threat in your bedroom is probably stubbing your toe on the way to the bathroom. But Steve doesn't know that. Steve is still scanning for saber-toothed tigers.

This is why logical approaches fail. You can't reason with Steve. You can't convince him with sheep counting. He's not operating from your rational mind—he's deep in your nervous system, running on instinct.

WHAT'S YOUR VERSION OF MIDNIGHT TORTURE?

- ❑ Mind that won't shut off
- ❑ Legs that won't stop moving
- ❑ Comfortable position you cannot find
- ❑ Temperature you can't regulate
- ❑ Sounds you can't stop hearing
- ❑ Worries you can't stop thinking

Patricia's 30-Year Midnight Marathon

Patricia dealt with Restless Leg Syndrome for three decades. Thirty years of her legs running their own midnight marathon while she desperately tried to sleep.

If you've never experienced RLS, imagine this: Just as you're drifting off, your legs decide to audition for the Rockettes. They twitch, ache, *demand* movement. The only relief is moving around or getting up and walking, which means . . . not sleeping.

Patricia tried everything medicine had to offer. She's in her late 70s, results-oriented, not interested in placebos or wishful thinking.

Then she decided to try Tapping.

After only a few times, 30 years of nightly torment resolved. Her restless leg syndrome was no longer an issue.

Patricia didn't just Interrupt a pattern; she demolished a three-decade Familiarity Trap. Her nervous system, which had been running the same program since she was in her 40s, Rewired itself in just a few sessions.

Her doctor was so impressed by her results—not just with sleep but with normalized thyroid numbers after Tapping—that Patricia got her primary care physician to try it himself.

Thirty years, Patricia suffered. How many years has it been for you?

THE SHIFT TO NEUROLOGICAL HYGIENE

We often wait until we are in a full-blown crisis, wide awake at 3 A.M. with our minds racing, to address our nervous system patterns. This is like waiting until you have 10 cavities to start brushing your teeth. To create lasting change with something like sleep, we need to move from emergency intervention to daily maintenance.

THE RULE:
Treat nervous system regulation like brushing your teeth–small, daily actions prevent major decay.

This concept of **Neurological Hygiene** is the key to deep, restorative sleep. Instead of only Tapping when you can't sleep, a short, five-minute Tapping session before bed can clear out the day's stress, calm the "security guard," and prepare your nervous system for rest. This proactive approach is often more powerful than an hour of reactive Tapping in the middle of the night.

The Biochemistry of the Bedroom Battlefield

Here's what's happening in your body during those sleepless nights, and why Tapping can flip the switch so dramatically:

- **The Cortisol Conspiracy:** When you can't sleep, cortisol (the stress hormone) starts rising. But here's the issue—cortisol is supposed to be at its lowest at night. It's like your body's internal clock is running on Tokyo time while you're in Tennessee.
- **The Melatonin Mutiny:** Your pineal gland should be pumping out melatonin (a sleep hormone) when darkness falls. But when your nervous system is in protection mode, melatonin production gets suppressed. Steve the Security Guard has overridden your natural sleep systems.
- **The Temperature Tango:** Your body temperature needs to drop for sleep to occur. But stress keeps your internal thermostat cranked up. It's like you're too hot-wired to sleep.
- **The Brainwave Rebellion:** Sleep requires your brainwaves to slow from active beta waves to relaxed alpha, then theta, then deep delta. But anxiety keeps you stuck in high-frequency beta, like trying to park a car while keeping the engine at full rev.

Tapping is the ultimate Pattern Interrupt for sleep issues, because it interrupts all these patterns simultaneously by sending specific neurochemical signals that reverse each of these sleep-blocking mechanisms. When you send those calming signals to your nervous system, you reduce cortisol and allow all other operations to return to a state of rest and digest—helping you ease into sleep naturally. Every tap is rewiring your biochemistry back to its natural sleep-wake cycle.

Susan's Sleep Study Surprise

Susan had been dependent on sleep medication for years. Not by choice, but by necessity. Without those pills, sleep simply didn't happen.

"I wanted to see if Tapping could replace it," she told us.

After a few months of nightly Tapping, she was medication-free and sleeping as much as before.

But the real surprise was in the data her sleep tracker was analyzing: "I watched the quality of my sleep change, with more time in deep sleep. In addition, my resting heart rate dropped by a few beats a minute."

Susan had successfully Rewired her sleep patterns. But here's where her story gets really interesting . . .

After a year, she got a little bored with her usual Tapping meditations and tried switching to regular sleep meditations. No Tapping, just standard relaxation meditations for sleep.

The result? Her deep sleep decreased. Her sleep quality declined.

"So last night I went back to your Tapping app. Boom. An hour and 40 minutes of deep sleep."

The fitness tracker doesn't lie. It doesn't know what meditation she's using. It just measures what's happening in her body. And what it measured was this: Tapping creates physiological changes that traditional meditation alone doesn't achieve.

In Susan's words, "The Fitbit has no skin in this game, so I'm guessing the difference is real."

THE DEAL YOU'VE MADE

What have you just "accepted" to be true for you?

Maybe you've accepted that . . .

- Good sleep is for other people
- You'll always be tired
- This is just how you're wired
- Nothing really works anyway
- Sleep is always going to be a struggle

When did you sign that contract? And are you ready to renegotiate the deal?

The Desperate Parent's Last Resort

Shauna's daughter Olivia didn't sleep for the first two years of her life.

Two. Years.

"She was awake five, six, seven times a night, every night!"

Any parent reading this just felt their soul leave their body. That's 730 nights of broken sleep. That's over 4,000 wake-ups. That's a level of exhaustion that threatens sanity, marriage, the will to live.

The doctor's solution? Antihistamines. Drug the baby to sleep.

"Even though I was at my wit's end and would have given my right arm for a night's sleep, the thought of medicating her didn't sit well with me."

In desperation, Shauna found an EFT practitioner who taught her to tap on Olivia.

"Within two to three nights of using it on her, she was sleeping through the night! It was like a miracle."

This story changed Shauna's entire life trajectory. She went on to have two more children ("who never would have been born if we hadn't found EFT for Olivia"), became an EFT Master Practitioner, and now helps others discover what saved her family.

This is what Tapping is all about. It's about interrupting a pattern that is prohibiting you from living your life (years of no sleep), and opening up an entirely new future. With Tapping, Shauna's entire family was transformed—two more lives and an entire career were created because of that one change.

The Revelation Hidden in Plain Night

Here's what took me years to fully understand about insomnia:

It's not a *sleep* problem. It's a *safety* problem.

Your body knows how to sleep. You did it as a baby (unless you were Olivia). The mechanism isn't broken. But somewhere along the way, your nervous system decided that staying awake was safer than sleeping.

This is the ultimate Familiarity Trap; your nervous system prefers the familiar discomfort of insomnia to the vulnerable uncertainty of sleep.

Maybe it started during a stressful period when you needed to be hypervigilant. Maybe it began after a trauma when your guard went up and never came down. Maybe it developed slowly as life's pressures accumulated.

The origin doesn't matter as much as the pattern: Your nervous system now treats bedtime as a threat rather than a respite.

This is why the words of a woman named Christine resonate so deeply: "For years, I struggled with getting a good night's sleep. My mind would race, my body felt tense, and falling asleep felt like a battle."

Falling asleep can feel like a battle because it *is* a battle—between the part of you that desperately needs rest and the part that's desperately trying to keep you safe by keeping you awake.

Every night, Christine hit the same Choice Point. Every night, she chose the familiar battle. Until she discovered she could Interrupt the war entirely.

As she told us later:

"At first I was hesitant and thought it was weird, but now I can honestly say it's been a game changer. I noticed big changes. I felt my body unwind as I tapped through my worries. The racing thoughts that used to keep me awake faded into the background. I now wake up feeling genuinely refreshed, which hasn't happened in years. Tapping has become a nightly routine for me."

PAUSE *and* REFLECT

Think back–when did sleep stop being easy? When did your system stop feeling safe enough to rest?

- During a stressful life period? (When: ______________________________)
- After a specific event? (What: ______________________________)
- Gradually over time? (Started noticing: ______________________________)
- Can't remember ever sleeping well? (Since:______________________________)

Your Sleep Sanctuary Awaits

Right now, as you read this, you might be thinking about tonight. That familiar dread might be creeping in—the preview of another wrestling match with your pillow, another staring contest with the ceiling.

Your inner Steve is already preparing for his shift, reviewing his list of everything that could go wrong if you dare close your eyes.

But here's what I want you to know: You're about to hit a Choice Point. The same one John faced. The same one Patricia encountered. The same one that changed Shauna's entire family's future.

You can choose another night of the same exhausting battle. Or you can choose to Interrupt the pattern and Rewire your relationship with sleep.

You see, Steve can be retrained. That hypervigilant security guard can learn that the night shift doesn't require constant alertness. Your nervous system can remember that darkness means rest, not danger.

John knows this now; he falls asleep so fast he can't finish the Tapping process. Patricia's legs rest peacefully after three decades of midnight marathons. Susan's deep sleep returned the moment she returned to Tapping. Shauna's daughter discovered what two years of life had hidden—the ability to sleep through the night.

They didn't develop better sleep hygiene. They didn't force themselves to relax. They didn't overcome their insomnia through willpower or fancy tricks.

They simply Recognized their pattern, Interrupted it with Tapping, and Rewired their nervous systems' fundamental approach to sleep.

What would you do with all the energy you currently spend dreading bedtime?

RECLAIMING *Your* FREEDOMS

The pattern we explored in this chapter doesn't just cause discomfort; it actively steals some of your 7 Freedoms. By using Tapping to rewire this pattern, you're not just getting rid of a problem–you're reclaiming your birthright to a full, vibrant life.

Take a moment to reflect: Which of these freedoms would open up the most for you if this pattern no longer had a hold on you?

- The freedom to experience emotions without being overwhelmed.
- The freedom to respond with wisdom instead of reacting from old wounds.
- The freedom to feel calm in situations that used to throw you.
- The freedom to access energy you didn't know you had.
- The freedom to feel at home and peaceful in your body.
- The freedom to trust yourself to handle whatever comes your way.
- The freedom to show up as your real self, not who you've been conditioned to be.

What is the first thing you would do, create, or experience with this newfound freedom?

Tonight's Different

Before long, tonight, you'll be in bed. Same bed. Same darkness. Same you.

But will it be the same pattern?

Or will tonight be the night you finally tell Steve his shift is over?

Feel that tiny spark of hope? That "maybe tonight could be different" feeling?

That's your nervous system ready to learn something new.

So here's my invitation:

Tonight, when you lay your head on that pillow, instead of beginning the usual negotiations, try something different.

Instead of fighting the situation, try making friends with the part of you that's keeping you awake. Thank Steve for his dedication. Let him know you appreciate his protection. Then gently show him that the night shift has been restructured. He can clock out. You've got this covered.

The sheep are exhausted from being counted. The ceiling is tired of being stared at. Your pillow is begging for a break from being flipped.

And you? You're ready to finally, actually sleep.

Because tonight, you're not going to force sleep. You're going to invite it. You're going to speak directly to your nervous system in the language it understands—gentle, rhythmic, bilateral stimulation that says, "All is well. You can rest now."

Your bed is waiting. Not as a battlefield, but as a sanctuary. Not as a place where old patterns rule, but as a space for new possibilities.

Ready to join the sleep revolution?

Let's tap.

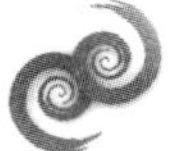

TAPPING SCRIPT: *Deep Sleep Portal*

Note: We recommend saving this meditation to do before bed when you are ready to fall asleep.

Let's check in.

On a scale of 0 to 10, how restless do you feel now? 10 is "wired and restless," and 0 is "relaxed and ready for sleep."

Take a gentle breath in . . . and out.

Start tapping on the side of your hand. Repeat either in your mind or out loud.

Side of the Hand: Even though my mind and body have trouble winding down, I acknowledge myself and my experience.

Even though I get frustrated when I can't sleep, I choose to be gentle with myself in this moment.

Even though part of me stays alert, I'm teaching my nervous system it's safe to relax.

Eyebrow: It can be hard to wind down
Side of the Eye: Sometimes it's just hard to let go of the day
Under the Eye: My mind is still so active
Under the Nose: My body feels restless
Under the Mouth: This desire to rest peacefully
Collarbone: Worrying about not getting enough rest
Under the Arm: This part of me that's on alert
Top of the Head: It just won't let me let go

Eyebrow: This part of me is trying to help
Side of the Eye: It's just trying to keep me safe
Under the Eye: But it's okay to stand down now
Under the Nose: Giving myself permission to rest
Under the Mouth: There's nothing to figure out right now
Collarbone: Nowhere to go and nothing to do
Under the Arm: It's okay to lower my guard
Top of the Head: It's safe to rest

Eyebrow: The day is done
Side of the Eye: I am safe in my bed
Under the Eye: My mind can begin to slow down
Under the Nose: My body can begin to settle
Under the Mouth: I don't have to force it
Collarbone: Just inviting rest into this moment
Under the Arm: It is safe to let go completely
Top of the Head: Winding down even more

Eyebrow:	Releasing any excess tension
Side of the Eye:	Allowing my muscles to soften . . .
Under the Eye:	and my breath to deepen
Under the Nose:	Feeling supported by the surface beneath me
Under the Mouth:	Feeling calmer with every breath
Collarbone:	Slowing down even more
Under the Arm:	I am safe
Top of the Head:	Safe to drift into deep sleep

Gently stop tapping and let your hands rest. Take a deep breath in . . . and let it out slowly.

How restless do you feel now on the 0-to-10 scale? If you feel more relaxed and sleepy, your new number will be lower.

Notice any shifts in your body. A yawn, a deeper breath, a sense of heaviness. Those are signs your nervous system is getting the message that it's safe to rest.

For a guided audio version of this Tapping meditation, visit www.thetappingsolution.com/rewired.

To Remember . . .

The Core Insight: *Insomnia is rarely a sleep problem; it's a safety problem. Your nervous system has learned to treat the vulnerability of sleep as a threat, keeping you on high alert. The hopeful truth is that you can retrain your body to recognize that your bed is a sanctuary, not a battlefield—so sleep can return naturally.*

The Practice: *Stop fighting for sleep, which only creates more alertness. Your practice is instead to create as much safety as you can—so sleep can. Use Tapping before bed as "neurological hygiene" to clear the day's stress. If you wake in the night, tap on your anxiety about not sleeping. Tap throughout the day to create a new baseline of ease. This is how you gently show your internal security guard that it is safe to stand down.*

CHAPTER 14

When Your Body Doesn't Feel Right

Easing Pain and Physical Symptoms

You already know from Chapter 1 how I discovered Tapping. It was a spring day in 2004 when a debilitating neck pain vanished in minutes. What I didn't tell you was how that experience messed with my head for months afterward.

I'd wake up every morning and carefully turn my neck, testing. Still no pain. I'd do it again at lunch. Before bed. Like a skeptic checking if a magic trick was still working.

The pain never came back, but something else did. A question that wouldn't leave me alone: If Tapping could eliminate physical pain that medications couldn't touch, what else were we getting wrong about our bodies?

What I didn't realize then was that I'd stumbled onto a way to interrupt a Reactive Loop—one of those automatic stress responses that fire without permission. My neck pain wasn't just physical; it was my nervous system's outdated alarm system, stuck in the "on" position.

Symptoms That Break All the Rules

Here's a statistic that should make you question everything: Up to 40 percent of people with herniated discs have zero pain. None. They only discover the bulging discs when getting MRIs for other reasons.

Same structural "damage." Completely different experience.

And then there's one of the most bizarre, and ultimately hope-filled, discoveries in all of neuroscience: the very real phenomenon of Phantom Limb Pain.

Imagine the confusion of a soldier who has lost a leg in battle but can feel an excruciating, itching, undeniable pain in a foot that is *no longer there.* For years, this was dismissed as being "all in their head." But we now know it is a real neurological event.

For decades, this phenomenon baffled science. But it has given us the ultimate proof of a life-changing truth: Many of our physical symptoms do not live exclusively in our body parts. They live in our brain's *map* of our body, in the stories and signals our nervous system has learned to run on repeat as Reactive Loops.

And this isn't just about amputated limbs or even chronic pain. This principle is the key to understanding a huge range of physical issues—the digestive problems that flare up under stress, the exhaustion that feels like a physical weight, the tension headaches that appear out of nowhere.

These are, in a sense, phantom symptoms for an emotional or stressful event that has already passed.

Gary's 15 Years of Pain

Gary, a veteran, had been living with back pain for 15 years. His MRI showed three bulging discs, clear evidence of why he hurt.

He'd tried everything he could think of that made sense for structural damage. The logic was sound: Fix the structure, fix the pain. Except nothing was working.

Eventually, a pain clinic recommended doing an ablation, a procedure where you burn off the nerves where the problem is, as a last resort. The first time they did that, it lasted about three months. But then the pain came back really, really bad. He had a second ablation done. Again, it provided temporary, minor relief. But life was still full of pain. Bend over too far, pain. Play golf, suffer for a few days after.

Over time, it just got worse, until life was unbearable. At this point, he could barely stand up, could barely walk across a parking lot without landing on the ground. When speaking to Jessica about this time in his life, she could hear the emotion get stuck in his throat. It wasn't just the pain. It was loss of freedom, loss of comfort, loss of life.

He was about to do another ablation procedure as a last resort when his wife mentioned that she'd been reading about "this Tapping thing."

In his words, Gary thought, "Oh, what the heck, I'll give it a try. So that's what I did."

At 72 years old, skeptical but desperate, Gary hit his Choice Point. He could continue the familiar path of medical procedures, or he could try something completely different. He went to his computer and looked up Tapping. He found a free Tapping meditation on our website, and gave it a try.

"Right away, I went from pain level 8 to a 1. Three days later . . . TOTALLY GONE!! I kept getting up, walking around and twisting and doing all kinds of stuff and kept telling my wife, you know, it's gone!"

The bulging discs didn't disappear. But after 15 years, his pain did. Why? Because he'd finally addressed the real issue—not the structural damage, but his nervous system's Reactive Loop.

He now taps every day with his wife, "Just because I know I feel better for doing it. I find, as does my wife, that I'm calmer and much more patient and tolerant than I used to be."

The story didn't stop there. Gary had a navy buddy who had been shot in the back in a hunting accident, and the bullet wedged in his spine left him with a lot of pain afterward.

The pain had kept him from sleeping well since the accident. Gary, encouraged by his own success, suggested his friend give Tapping a try.

His friend was skeptical, but he tried it. And the relief it offered him was palpable. He told Gary that the very first night he tried it, he was able to sleep without pain keeping him up.

Although his friend still experiences pain from the wound, Tapping helps lower the pain enough that he can now rest each night, which leads to a massive shift in quality of life. And so he taps every single night.

How long have you been living with your body's struggles? When did you stop counting in months and start counting in years? When did "managing symptoms" become your second job?

The Neuroscience of Pain Loops

- **The Pain–Stress Cycle**
  - Chronic pain triggers stress hormones (like cortisol and adrenaline).
  - Stress increases inflammation and muscle tension, which feeds back into more pain.
  - Over time, the amygdala (the brain's alarm center) becomes hypersensitive to body signals, amplifying the pain experience.
- **Neural Pathway Reinforcement**
  - Every repetition of pain strengthens the brain's pain circuits through neuroplasticity.
  - It's like water carving grooves in rock—after years, those grooves become canyons.
  - The result: Pain feels automatic and hard to escape.
- **The Expectation Effect**
  - fMRI studies show that anticipating pain activates brain pain centers even before movement or injury.
  - Gary's brain was generating pain simply from the fear and expectation of movement.
- **How Tapping Interrupts the Loop**
  - Focusing on pain acknowledges the signal (exposure).
  - Tapping on acupressure points sends calming, safety signals to the amygdala and nervous system.
  - This "dual input" helps the brain reassess the threat, weaken the old Reactive Loop, and begin rewiring for relief.

The Slow Surrender: The Life You've Stopped Living

Let's pause for a moment. Before we dive into why your body's doing what it's doing, I want you to take inventory of something you might not have noticed happening.

What have you stopped doing because of how your body feels?

Really think about it. Not the obvious stuff like "I don't run marathons anymore." I mean the small surrenders. The tiny negotiations. The gradual shrinking of your world.

Maybe you:

- Don't sit on the floor or certain chairs anymore because getting back up hurts too much
- Turn down dinner invitations because certain foods trigger reactions
- Carry antihistamines everywhere "just in case"
- Sleep in that one specific position that doesn't make things worse
- Schedule your entire day around your energy crashes
- Plan trips around your safe foods and familiar bathrooms
- Say "I'm tired" when people ask how you are—every single time

Maybe your body has slowly, quietly, trained you to play smaller.

And here's the sneaky part: It often happens so gradually we don't even notice. Each accommodation seems reasonable at the time. "Oh, I'll just avoid that." "I'll just be careful." "I'll just rest first."

Just. Just. Just.

Each "just" is our world getting a little smaller.

Each "just" is you falling deeper into a Familiarity Trap—choosing the familiar limitation over the unknown possibility of freedom.

Take a moment right now. What does your body stop you from doing? What everyday pleasures have you quietly removed from your life?

Got your list? Feel that weight of all you've given up?

Good. Because here's what I need you to understand: Your body hasn't betrayed you. It's not broken. It's not falling apart.

It's just confused about danger versus safety. It just doesn't quite understand that danger is over.

And shifting that is how everything changes.

Why Your Body Is Basically a (Bad) Alarm System That's Stuck in the "On" Position

Here's the simplest way to understand what's happening in your body right now:

Your nervous system is like an alarm system. When it detects danger, real or imagined, it sounds various alarms:

- Pain (pay attention here!)
- Muscle tension (prepare to run!)
- Inflammation (mobilize defenses!)
- Digestive issues (no time for food processing!)
- High blood pressure (pump resources faster!)

Brilliant design for actual danger. It screams when there's smoke, you escape the fire, everyone survives.

Terrible design for modern life when your nervous system can't tell the difference between a looming deadline and a tiger chasing you in the woods.

In this modern lifestyle we're living, our systems are stuck screaming about:

- The e-mail that felt threatening (but wasn't)
- The deadline that felt life-or-death (but wasn't)
- The conflict that felt dangerous (but wasn't)
- The painful memory that feels like current reality (but isn't)

Our bodies are like smoke detectors that get stuck in the "on" position. Sometimes, they keep screaming about a fire that was extinguished years ago.

The medical approach? Try to muffle the alarm with medications. Or surgically disconnect it. Or cover it up with other things.

But what if you could simply remind the system that the danger has passed? Or that whatever it's wailing about isn't actually so dangerous after all?

QUICK CHECK: READING YOUR BODY'S ALARMS

Right now, scan your body from head to toe:

- Where do you feel tension?
- What areas feel "loud" or demand attention?
- If this sensation had a message, what would it be?
- What might your body be trying to protect you from?

Reflect on or write down your first instinct. Often our initial response reveals more than we think.

Why This Changes Everything

When I had that neck pain in 2004, every medical professional would have had the same advice:

- Rest
- Ice/heat
- Anti-inflammatories
- Muscle relaxers
- If it persists, get an MRI

They would have looked for structural problems. They would have treated the physical symptoms. And they would have missed the entire point.

Because my neck wasn't broken. My nervous system was stuck in alarm mode.

The Migraines That (Used to) Run in the Family

Maní grew up watching her mother struggle with debilitating migraines. Whenever stress and overwhelm hit—and in their chaotic household, it hit often—her mother would be knocked out by crushing migraines that lasted for days.

Maní thought she'd escaped that particular inheritance. Then she became a mother herself.

Suddenly, the same pattern emerged, and the migraines set in. For 20 years, she found herself living the same story: stress building up until her body sounded the alarm and shut down with blinding pain. The migraines began to run her entire life.

But Maní decided that pattern would stop with her.

She found the Tapping app and started simple: the anxiety meditation when she felt overwhelmed, the anger meditation when frustration built. "Just those two got me 70 percent of my results," she said.

The transformation was remarkable. A month passed, and she realized she hadn't had a migraine. Another month, no migraine.

What was once a common occurrence is now a rare occasion. She shared that now, if a migraine does show up, she's able to hear the alarm, soothe it with Tapping, and stop the migraine in its tracks so it's not debilitating her for an entire day.

Five years and 5,000 Tapping sessions later, Maní hasn't just freed herself from migraines. She's broken a generational pattern of women whose bodies translated stress into crushing pain.

She Recognized the inherited Reactive Loop, Interrupted it with Tapping, and created a Rewired Response where stress no longer triggers debilitating pain.

THE PARADOX OF ACKNOWLEDGMENT: THE "TELL THE TRUTH" RULE

Our instinct is often to push pain (physical or emotional) away, to ignore it, or to immediately try to force a positive state. Tapping works on a completely different principle. To release a symptom or emotion, you must first be willing to fully and honestly acknowledge its presence.

THE RULE:
What you resist, persists. What you acknowledge (while tapping), releases.

The Tapping process only works when you tell the radical truth about how you feel and what you're experiencing *right now*. When you start your Tapping sequence by saying, "This throbbing pain in my head," or "This deep ache in my lower back," you aren't "dwelling on the negative." You are shining a spotlight on the precise pattern your nervous system needs to address.

Acknowledging the truth while you tap is what allows your nervous system to finally stand down its alarm, neutralizing the charge and creating space for relief.

The Question That Could Change Your Life

Right now, you might be living with something—a pain, a symptom—that you've been told is just "how things are." Maybe you've had it so long it feels like part of your identity. "I'm the person with the bad back/migraines/allergies."

Let's get specific about *your* normal:

- "I always get headaches when . . ."
- "My stomach acts up every time . . ."
- "My back goes out when . . ."
- "I'm exhausted after . . ."
- "I react badly to . . ."

Read those statements. How many times have you said them? How many times have you accepted them as facts instead of changeable patterns?

And what if that identity is based on a misunderstanding?

What if your body isn't broken, it's just stuck in alarm mode?

What if the symptom that seems so permanent is actually your nervous system's changeable response to an old threat?

Every time you tap while focusing on physical discomfort, you're essentially having this conversation with your nervous system:

"Hey, I know you're trying to protect me by creating this [insert pain or symptom]. I appreciate your dedication. But the danger you're responding to? It's over. You can stand down now."

If your most bothersome symptom improved by just 30 percent, what would that free you up to do? How would your days change? What choices would become available?

The Tapping Teacher Who Forgets to Tap

Here's something I want to confess: Sometimes I'll walk around with a crick in my neck for hours before remembering I could tap it away in minutes.

Yes, me. The guy who discovered Tapping because of neck pain in 2004. The person who's taught millions to tap for physical symptoms. Just . . . living with unnecessary pain because I forgot to use my own tool. Even after 20 years, I sometimes choose the Familiarity Trap of "just dealing with it" over taking two minutes to Interrupt the pattern.

Why? Because Reactive Loops are sneaky. They feel normal. They feel like "just how things are." Breaking them requires conscious choice—hitting that Choice Point and actively choosing something different.

Like last week at midnight, when I woke up with my throat on fire. Did I immediately tap? No. I lay there for five minutes feeling sorry for myself until my brain finally kicked in: "Wait, you actually teach this for a living."

Five minutes of Tapping. Sore throat melted away just enough that I could sleep peacefully. And I'm lying there in the dark thinking, "How does this STILL shock me after twenty years?"

I share this because if you've ever known *exactly* what would help but didn't do it anyway, you're in good company. Sometimes (okay, most of the time), it feels easier to just pop an Advil or wait it out or sit there in agony complaining about it.

We all sometimes choose familiar suffering over unfamiliar solutions, even when we *know* there's an option we could try that works.

I think about Tapping all day long and I've made a whole career out of it. And yet, I'm not the perfect teacher who immediately addresses every symptom. I'm the imperfect human who sometimes needs to hurt for a while before remembering I don't have to.

But when I do remember? It works. Every time.

A Demo That Reminds Us Why We Do What We Do

Sometimes the most powerful healings happen when we least expect them. Alex once told me about a demonstration at a local health food store that reminded him why we do this work.

He was there doing a Tapping demo, one of those informal gatherings where curious people stop by to learn about this "weird technique." A woman approached who hadn't been able to raise her arm properly in 20 years. Twenty years of limited movement (I'm talking just barely being able to raise it), of adapting her entire life around this limitation.

Can you imagine what that would be like? Two decades of not being able to reach the top shelf. Of struggling to put on certain clothes. Of that constant reminder every time she tried to lift something that her body had these borders, these no-go zones.

In just 15 minutes of tapping together, this woman raised her arm above her head.

This wasn't a miracle cure or magic. It was simply what happens when a nervous system that's been bracing for two decades finally gets the message that it's safe to let go. When the alarm that's been blaring for what seems like forever finally gets turned off.

Stories like these happen every day in our community. Because so many of our physical limitations aren't actually physical—they're our nervous system's outdated protection programs still running long after the danger has passed.

RECLAIMING *Your* FREEDOMS

The pattern we explored in this chapter doesn't just cause discomfort; it actively steals some of your 7 Freedoms. By using Tapping to rewire this pattern, you're not just getting rid of a problem–you're reclaiming your birthright to a full, vibrant life.

Take a moment to reflect: Which of these freedoms would open up the most for you if this pattern no longer had a hold on you?

- The freedom to experience emotions without being overwhelmed.
- The freedom to respond with wisdom instead of reacting from old wounds.
- The freedom to feel calm in situations that used to throw you.
- The freedom to access energy you didn't know you had.
- The freedom to feel at home and peaceful in your body.
- The freedom to trust yourself to handle whatever comes your way.
- The freedom to show up as your real self, not who you've been conditioned to be.

What is the first thing you would do, create, or experience with this newfound freedom?

Your Body's Resignation Letter

If your body could write you a letter, it might say: "I've been on high alert for so long, I forgot what normal feels like. I've been protecting you from dangers that passed years ago. I'm exhausted from sounding alarms nobody turns off. I'm ready to remember what wellness feels like. Are you?"

The Choice Point You Face Right Now

Every person in this chapter faced the same Choice Point you're facing:

Keep treating the physical symptoms while your nervous system stays in alarm mode or finally address the alarm itself.

Gary could have had more ablations. I could have taken a painkiller for my neck. Maní could have run through the list of migraine medications available to her.

Instead, we chose to ask a different question: What if my body's not broken? What if it's just scared?

We chose to speak to our nervous systems in the language of safety, through Tapping, rather than trying to force change through willpower or medical interventions.

And our bodies responded by doing what bodies do when they feel safe: They healed.

The Permission Your Body's Been Waiting For

As I write this, 20 years after that neck pain changed my life, I'm still amazed by the pattern:

Physical symptom appears → Person tries everything to address the symptom → Nothing fully works → They try Tapping → They finally address the issue at the nervous system level → Symptom resolves

Not because Tapping is magic. But because it finally addresses what's actually happening: a nervous system stuck in protective mode, creating symptoms to keep you vigilant about a danger that either isn't so dangerous after all or no longer exists in the present moment.

One last check-in. That thing your body does—the pain, the reaction, the exhaustion, the sensitivity—what if it's not permanent? What if it's not "just how you are"? What if it's just your nervous system's way of trying to keep you safe from something that's already over?

Feel that possibility? Even just a crack of hope? That's all we need.

Because in the next few minutes, you're going to have a conversation with your body you've never had before. You're going to thank it for protecting you. Then you're going to gently let it know the war is over.

Your body has been loyally protecting you, maybe for years or decades. Isn't it time to gently turn off the alarm?

Your healing might be dramatic and instant, or it might be gradual and subtle. Both are victories. Both are your nervous system learning it's safe to let go. Both are you reclaiming your life, one tap at a time.

Ready to sound the all-clear?

Let's tap.

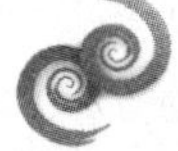

TAPPING SCRIPT:
Support Your Body: Relax and Restore

Let's start by checking in with your body.

Tune in to any physical discomfort, tension, or unease you're feeling. On a scale of 0 to 10, how intense is that sensation? 10 is "very intense"; 0 is "completely calm and at ease."

Take a gentle breath in . . . and out.

Start tapping on the side of your hand. Repeat either in your mind or out loud.

Side of the Hand: Even though my body is holding on to some discomfort,
and I wish I felt more at ease,
I choose to tune in with compassion.

Even though I get frustrated with physical symptoms,
and I just want them to go away,
I honor my body for working so hard for me.

Even though my body sometimes sounds alarms,
I'm open to reminding my nervous system that I am safe.

Eyebrow: This physical discomfort
Side of the Eye: This struggle with my body
Under the Eye: I'm tired of not feeling good
Under the Nose: I've been so frustrated with my body
Under the Mouth: It's easy to lose trust in it
Collarbone: I feel like I'm battling my body
Under the Arm: I acknowledge all these feelings . . .
Top of the Head: and recognize my own unique struggles

Eyebrow: My body has been on high alert
Side of the Eye: Experiencing so much stress
Under the Eye: It's been trying to protect me
Under the Nose: I now tune in and listen
Under the Mouth: I reassure my body it is safe
Collarbone: Going from fight or flight . . .
Under the Arm: to heal and restore
Top of the Head: It is safe for my mind and body to rest

Eyebrow: Safety is where healing begins . . .
Side of the Eye: and my body knows what to do
Under the Eye: Welcoming deep comfort . . .
Under the Nose: and greater ease
Under the Mouth: Creating a space for healing
Collarbone: Supporting my body . . .
Under the Arm: through my loving words and actions
Top of the Head: I'm a good friend to my body

Eyebrow: Feeling a new respect for my body
Side of the Eye: Letting my body know it's safe
Under the Eye: Safe to soften . . .
Under the Nose: safe to let go . . .
Under the Mouth: safe to recover
Collarbone: Opening up to more ease
Under the Arm: Allowing healing to happen
Top of the Head: My body can rest

Gently stop tapping and let your hands rest. Take a deep breath in . . . and let it out slowly.

Check back in with that physical sensation. Where is the intensity on the 0-to-10 scale now? Even a small shift is proof that you can change the signals your body is sending.

Your body has been protecting you the only way it knows how. Now it's time to update the system. Time to remember what it feels like to be well.

For a guided audio version of this Tapping meditation, visit www.thetappingsolution.com/rewired.

To Remember . . .

The Core Insight: *Many physical symptoms are alarm signals from a nervous system stuck in a state of threat. But your body knows how to feel better. Your power lies in your ability to turn off the constant alarm bells so your body's natural healing intelligence can do its work.*

The Practice: *Your practice is to acknowledge the physical symptom with honesty while you tap. Use phrases like "this throbbing pain" or "this tightness in my gut." This shines a spotlight on the specific pattern. At the same time, the act of tapping sends a signal of safety that allows your nervous system to stand down its alarm, creating the conditions for relief.*

CHAPTER 15

When You Face a Health Challenge

Activating Your Natural Healing Abilities

Here's what 20 years of watching people tap away "permanent" health problems has taught me:

Your body doesn't know the difference between emotional danger and physical danger. To your nervous system, they're the same threat requiring the same Reactive Loop: SOUND THE ALARM.

We explored this in the last chapter with those everyday symptoms that become our unwanted companions: the neck pain, the migraines, the backaches that seem so permanent until they suddenly aren't.

But the mind-body connection goes even deeper than that, and nobody explains that to us.

Sometimes we find ourselves with blood pressure readings that won't budge, complex diagnoses, or conditions that have you reorganizing your entire life around doctor's appointments and treatment protocols.

The fascinating part is that even with these more complex health situations, the mind-body connection is still at play.

Think about it:

- Betrayal feels like a punch to the gut and can cause gut issues
- Heartbreak feels like chest pain and can cause actual chest pain
- Carrying the weight of the world causes shoulder/back pain
- Being "fed up" creates digestive problems

This isn't metaphorical. It's measurable neuroscience. When you experience emotional stress, your hypothalamic-pituitary-adrenal (HPA) axis activates the same cascade of stress hormones as if you were facing physical danger. Your body can't tell the difference between heartbreak and a heart-attack threat.

The Blood Pressure Proof

Eugene discovered this mind-body connection in the most measurable way possible. Sitting with his blood pressure monitor, his reading showed the usual high numbers: above 130/77.

Instead of deep breathing or meditating, he did something that felt more intuitive to him.

Feeling a heaviness and pressure in his heart, he started tapping while focusing on his heart. And as he tapped, he let his mind wander, and he noticed old memories and feelings come up.

He felt tension build up in his body as all these feelings showed up, but he stuck with it. And eventually, he was surprised by the shift that occurred, the feeling of lightness and release.

What was interesting was that his body reflected the emotional experience he just had. After he finished tapping, he checked the blood pressure monitor again: 101/77.

Five minutes of Tapping. A 30-point drop. A reflection that the inner work has physical manifestations that can be scientifically measured.

This story shows us just how our bodies are capable of translating emotional experiences into physical conditions. It's not "all in your head"—it's in your body because your head put it there. And sometimes, this connection shows up not just as aches and pains, but as major health challenges and diagnoses that change everything.

When Cancer Came Knocking: Elizabeth's Story

Elizabeth was 67 when the diagnosis arrived, right before Christmas. Cancer. The word that changes everything.

"I wasn't ready to tell my family," she shared with Jessica.

As she processed the news internally, she turned to Tapping. Not to cure her cancer, but to find solid ground in a world that had suddenly tilted off its axis.

What she discovered changed her entire cancer journey. Instead of bouncing between panic and denial (the two places most of us land with terrifying diagnoses), Tapping helped her find a third option: centered presence.

"In that calm space, I could actually think," Elizabeth explained. "I could be creative about finding support. I could advocate for myself with doctors."

She continued to explain that when you have a diagnosis like cancer, you often have to make decisions with little information, not knowing which path is the best to take, with no guarantees either way. Tapping helped her tune in to what felt best for her, so she could make those decisions.

The most remarkable moment came during chemotherapy. The protocol called for 12 sessions, but by session 7, Elizabeth's body was screaming for a break. Not quitting, just pausing.

Through Tapping, she'd learned to distinguish between fear and wisdom. She spoke up and asked her doctors for a break. And they agreed.

During that pause, the scans came back: No detectable cancer. Four weeks later, still clear. She completed the full 12 sessions for extra certainty, but that intuition-guided pause gave her body just what it needed: time to recover before the treatments resumed.

Today, Elizabeth is cancer-free. Not because Tapping cured her cancer; it didn't. But because it gave her access to the wisdom, clarity, and sense of self-empowerment she needed to navigate her treatment program successfully.

Tapping isn't a miracle cure-all. It's not just about making symptoms disappear and feeling better after a session or two.

Sometimes its truest, most profound power is helping you find peace in the storm long enough to make the decisions that lead to healing.

The Invitation Within the Challenge

The moment you receive a serious health diagnosis, two journeys begin. The first is external: a path of doctors, treatments, and tests. The second journey is internal: a path of navigating fear, finding strength, and redefining hope. While the first is guided by medical experts, the second is one you must walk yourself. But you don't have to walk it without a map.

A health challenge, as difficult as it is, can also be an invitation. It's an invitation to connect with a depth of resilience you never knew you had. An invitation to listen to your body with a new level of compassion. And an invitation to discover that you have far more influence over your inner world—your peace, your clarity, and your hope—than you've ever been led to believe.

The Science of Healing States

- **Stress Mode vs. Healing Mode**
    - In **stress mode** (sympathetic dominance), your body prioritizes survival: racing heart, tense muscles, shallow breath.
    - In **healing mode** (parasympathetic dominance), resources shift to repair, digestion, and immune defense.
- **How Stress Impacts Cells**
    - Chronic stress keeps you stuck in survival, leaving little energy for healing.
    - Elevated cortisol can weaken immunity, reduce natural killer cell activity, raise inflammation, and impair DNA repair.
    - Over time, this makes the body less able to recover and regenerate.
- **Why Calm Heals**
    - Finding calm isn't just mental, it's biological.
    - Shifting into healing mode signals safety to your body, allowing it to restore, repair, and strengthen.

Stress mode feels wired, tense, and exhausting, like you're bracing for impact. Healing mode feels slower, softer, more grounded; your breath deepens, your shoulders drop, and your body finally has space to repair itself.

Breaking Through the Great Forgetting: Your Body Already Knows How to Heal

We've forgotten something crucial about healing: Your body's natural state is health. It knows how to:

- Regulate blood pressure
- Relax muscles
- Reduce inflammation
- Digest properly
- Sleep deeply
- Heal wounds
- Regulate hormones
- Fight infections
- Repair and rebuild tissue

But these healing mechanisms go offline when you're stuck in stress-based Reactive Loops. Every moment spent in "This shouldn't be happening" or "I can't handle this" is a moment your body can't dedicate to healing.

Tapping doesn't cure disease. But it takes your nervous system out of alarm mode so your body can do what it's designed to do: heal. It's the difference between trying to repair a house while the fire alarm is blaring versus working in peaceful quiet.

Your Body's User Manual (The One Nobody Gave You)

Imagine if your body came with a user manual. Page one would say: *WARNING: This system is designed to prioritize survival over comfort. Physical healing accelerates dramatically once alarm mode is deactivated.*

That's what Tapping does. It doesn't promise to cure your illness; it promises to quiet the alarm so your body has the best possible internal environment to do what it's naturally designed to do: recover and heal.

Support, Not Substitution

Let me be absolutely clear about what Tapping can and cannot do:

Tapping CANNOT:

- Replace medical treatment
- Cure diseases through wishful thinking
- Make medications unnecessary at all times
- Fix a broken bone

Tapping CAN:

- Reduce treatment side effects
- Help you make clearer medical decisions
- Lower stress that impedes healing
- Release emotions stored in the body
- Restore hope and agency
- Support your body's innate healing capacity

Think of it this way: If your body is fighting a battle (against cancer, autoimmune conditions, chronic illness), Tapping helps you stop fighting a war on two fronts. It calms the internal stress response so your body can direct more resources toward healing.

The Truth About "Miraculous" Healings

Let me be clear about something: Not everyone's blood pressure will go down in one Tapping session. Not every case of chronic illness will vanish. Not everyone will have these same incredible results right away.

And that's okay.

What matters isn't the speed of healing; it's the idea that healing is possible at all.

Even shifting symptoms from a 10 to a 7 can be life-changing. Why? Because for every point you drop, you're adding something back to your life.

When you're at a 7 instead of a 10, you can think clearly enough to make different choices. At a 7, you might:

- Actually want to try that gentle yoga class
- Have energy to cook a healthy meal instead of ordering takeout
- Feel present enough to enjoy a conversation
- Sleep deeply enough to let your body repair itself

If that's possible at a 7, can you imagine what would be possible at a 5? Or a 3?

The gap between "complete agony" and "manageable discomfort," or between "overwhelming fear" and "concerned but coping" is where life happens.

Elizabeth didn't tap away her cancer. She tapped her way to clarity, which led to an empowering treatment decision.

This isn't about miraculous instant cures (though yes, those happen sometimes, and when they do, it's incredible). This is about giving your nervous system a new option besides screaming alarm bells. It's about creating enough calm in the storm that you can see the way forward.

THE 20% PRINCIPLE

Most of us are trapped in all-or-nothing thinking. We believe we need complete transformation before we can start living again—100 percent pain-free, completely healed, totally better. This perfectionism keeps us stuck, waiting for a miracle that may never come in the exact form we're imagining.

THE RULE:
You don't need perfect healing to reclaim your life.
A 20 percent improvement changes everything.

The 20 Percent Principle recognizes a profound truth: small shifts create cascading changes. When you're 20 percent less exhausted, you might take that walk. That walk improves your mood by 20 percent. That mood lift gives you 20 percent more patience with your family. That patience reduces relationship stress by 20 percent. And suddenly, your entire life is shifting—not because you're "cured," but because you're 20 percent better.

The Courage to Hope Again

Perhaps the cruelest part of chronic illness is how it steals hope. After enough failed treatments, disappointing appointments, and "learning to live with it" speeches, you stop believing things can change.

Tapping doesn't promise a cure. But it does offer this: the possibility that tomorrow could feel different from today.

Even if your condition remains, your experience of it can transform. And sometimes—not always, but sometimes—when the nervous system calms and the emotional charge releases, the body surprises everyone with what it can do.

Your Healing Team Needs You on It

For too long, we've been taught to see our bodies as machines to be fixed or enemies to be fought. A diagnosis can amplify this feeling, creating a painful disconnect from the very vessel we need to carry us through healing. Tapping offers a different path: partnership.

Think of healing like a team sport. You've got:

- Doctors (strategy)
- Medications/treatments (tools)
- Your body (the player)

But who's the coach? Who's calling plays based on deep knowledge of the player?

That's you. And Tapping helps you hear what your body needs so you can coach effectively.

Elizabeth knew her body needed a chemo break. And she knew it because Tapping quieted the noise enough for her to hear her inner wisdom.

Under all the fear, beneath the symptoms, beyond the diagnoses—your body's natural tendency is toward health. It just needs your support, direction, and love to help it remember it's safe.

Ready to find your calm and support your body?

Let's tap.

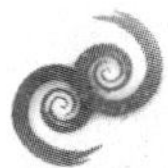

TAPPING SCRIPT: *Finding Ease Through a Health Challenge*

Let's start by checking in.

Acknowledge the worry, the fear, or the physical discomfort you're holding about your health. Rate the intensity of this feeling on a scale of 0 to 10, with 10 being you feel extremely stressed about your health challenges and 0 being you feel calm and centered.

Take a gentle breath in . . . and out.

Start tapping on the side of your hand. Repeat either in your mind or out loud.

Side of the Hand: Even though I sometimes worry about my health,
and it feels overwhelming,
I choose to be kind to myself right now.

Even though there is so much uncertainty,
and I feel this fear in my body,
there is space for all of my feelings.

Even though this is hard,
I'm open to finding a sense of ease in the middle of it all.

Eyebrow: All this worry about my health
Side of the Eye: This feeling of being overwhelmed
Under the Eye: All the "what ifs"
Under the Nose: This fear in my body
Under the Mouth: It's all so heavy
Collarbone: It's hard to know what to do
Under the Arm: All this uncertainty
Top of the Head: All this stress in my system

Eyebrow: But I am here now
Side of the Eye: Tapping and breathing
Under the Eye: Sending a signal of calm to my body
Under the Nose: Letting my nervous system know . . .
Under the Mouth: that in this moment, I am okay
Collarbone: It is safe to relax
Under the Arm: Releasing the need to control everything
Top of the Head: Allowing a sense of ease to wash over me

Eyebrow: When my mind and body are quiet . . .
Side of the Eye: it's easier to know what feels right for me
Under the Eye: I am beginning to find my way . . .
Under the Nose: with curiosity and creativity
Under the Mouth: Feeling capable and resourceful . . .
Collarbone: as I navigate this challenge
Under the Arm: I'm a powerful advocate for myself
Top of the Head: I direct my energy toward healing

Eyebrow: Empowering my body with hopeful thoughts
Side of the Eye: Supporting my body with loving actions
Under the Eye: I'm open to new possibilities
Under the Nose: Even in this body . . .
Under the Mouth: I can experience more joy and energy
Collarbone: I'm open to surprising myself
Under the Arm: I'm finding my way as I go
Top of the Head: Moving forward with hope and trust

Gently stop tapping and let your hands rest. Take a deep breath in . . . and let it out slowly . . .

How intense is that fear or stress about your health now, on the 0-to-10 scale?

Notice any shift, however small, toward peace. This is your power.

For a guided audio version of this Tapping meditation, visit www.thetappingsolution.com/rewired.

To Remember . . .

The Core Insight: *Tapping is not a replacement for medical care, but a powerful tool to support it. Its profound power lies in helping you find peace in the storm long enough to make clear decisions, advocate for yourself, and create an internal state that is optimal for healing.*

The Practice: *When facing a health challenge, tap on the emotional truth of your experience: the fear, the anger, the overwhelm. By acknowledging these feelings while sending calming signals to your nervous system, you create the inner space needed to navigate your journey with wisdom and resilience.*

CHAPTER 16

When Other People Drive You Crazy

Staying Centered No Matter Who Is Around

"I honestly can say that Tapping saved my marriage. I don't know how else to explain it."

That's how Donna describes what happened after 25 years of marriage nearly ended in divorce papers.

She and her husband had always had their differences, but this time was different. The fights had escalated beyond anything they'd experienced before. Every conversation became a minefield. Every interaction felt like a chess match where both players were trying to checkmate the other.

"We were at a different level," Donna explained. "I actually asked him to leave."

Have you ever experienced that before? When the person you're supposed to love most becomes the person who triggers you fastest?

When you find yourself stuck in the Familiarity Trap of having the same fight for the hundredth time, just with different words?

Donna was living in that hell. Until she hit her Choice Point. Instead of continuing down the familiar path toward divorce, she decided to Interrupt the pattern.

She started tapping. Just Donna, alone, tapping on her own reactions to her husband and the tense dynamic that had been created between them.

And then something extraordinary happened:

"I started responding differently to my husband . . . WITHOUT TRYING OR THINKING ABOUT IT! I mean I didn't react to certain things he said or didn't take offense or was able to have a normal conversation. It was so weird!"

Same husband. Same marriage. Same 25-year history of patterns. But suddenly, Donna was showing up differently. And when one person in a relationship changes their wiring, everything changes.

One year later, sitting with her husband, Donna realized something remarkable: "We had not had a fight or argument for twelve months! Twelve months!!!"

She asked him if he'd noticed the chance. His response? "That's funny cause I just mentioned to a friend that things have been going smoothly for about six months."

Donna had spent a full year rewiring her relationship patterns through Tapping, and her husband didn't even know she was doing it. He just knew their marriage had somehow become . . . peaceful.

From Sibling Rivalry to Family Business

Donna's story is a powerful testament to how one person can unilaterally change the dynamic of a romantic partnership. But this principle of rewiring extends beyond marriage. It can transform the most foundational and, at times, the most frustrating relationships of all: the ones we have with our family.

Growing up, Jessica, Alex, and I were typical siblings. We had our moments—the pranks, the occasional squabbles, the standard "Mom, he's bothering me!" car rides. Overall, we got along well. But like most families, we each developed our own emotional triggers that would follow us into adulthood.

And now, as you know, the three of us run The Tapping Solution business together, as a team.

Jessica recently shared something that perfectly illustrates how childhood patterns can hijack our adult relationships:

"Being the youngest sister of two older brothers, I often felt left out. I couldn't play basketball in our driveway—too young and short. Couldn't play Nintendo in our basement—there were only two remotes. So 'feeling left out' became an easy emotional trigger for me.

"Years later, when we started our business together, Nick and Alex had what felt to me like an important meeting, and I wasn't there. I was *so* angry. When the reality was it was just an organic conversation that happened to occur when I wasn't around. My emotional reaction didn't match the reality of the situation at all.

"I realized I needed to tap on my feelings of being left out. I'd held that with me from childhood, and my nervous system was stuck scanning for situations that I could interpret through that lens. This childhood Reactive Loop was still running my adult life."

This is the perfect example of how our nervous systems carry old programs into new situations. Jessica's brain was still protecting her from being the left-out little sister, even though she was now an equal, respected partner in our business.

We often joke that our family business is proof Tapping works, because nothing can trigger you like your own family! If we, three siblings, can run a business together with relative peace and harmony (no one's perfect), then there's got to be something to this whole Tapping thing.

Sure, we have our moments. We have disagreements. But we've each done the work to recognize our individual triggers and patterns. We've created a beautiful dynamic that allows each of us to play to our strengths while managing our old wounds.

Our journey from typical siblings to business partners encapsulates what "rewiring" on a relationship level actually looks like. The people who know exactly which buttons to push can become your greatest allies and partners—once you stop playing by the old rules and choose to interrupt the pattern.

The Invisible Tax on Your Peace

You might think this chapter is just about getting along better with people. It's not. This is about reclaiming the vast amounts of energy, mental space, and physical well-being that are being stolen by relationship friction every single day. Why should you care about this? Because tensions in your relationships with others are secretly eroding the core benefits we're working toward in this book:

- **Your Quieter Mind:** How much of your mental chatter is spent replaying conversations, anticipating conflicts, or cataloging other people's faults? Every ounce of energy spent on that inner commentary is energy not available for your own peace and creativity.

- **Peace in Your Body:** That familiar tension in your shoulders when your boss e-mails? The knot in your stomach when your partner is in a mood? That's your nervous system going into threat mode. Constant relationship friction keeps your body marinating in stress hormones, preventing it from ever feeling truly safe and at ease.
- **A Life of Possibility:** The energy you burn being annoyed at your co-worker is energy you can't put toward that passion project. The focus you lose fuming about your teenager is focus you can't give to your career. Your relationships are either a source of energy or a drain on it. Rewiring your reactions turns a drain into a fountain.

This relationship friction is part of the Great Forgetting. We are so used to tension and conflict and bickering and disconnection that we've forgotten what it feels like to stay centered and peaceful, even if people try to push our buttons or bring chaos to our lives.

This chapter is about stopping the leaks. It's about plugging the holes in your energy and peace that other people's behavior creates, not by changing them, but by changing your response.

YOUR RELATIONSHIP ENERGY AUDIT

Take a moment to honestly assess:

- Which relationship in your life drains the most energy right now?
- On a typical day, what percentage of your mental chatter is about this person's behavior or your interactions?
- If this dynamic continues unchanged for the next five years, what will it cost you? Your health? Your joy? Your other relationships?
- What would open up in your life if you could stay centered around this person?

Write down your answers. The clarity might surprise you.

The Emotional Debt You're Accumulating

Think of your relationships like a bank account. Every positive interaction is a deposit. Every difficult moment—every eye-roll, every broken promise, every bit of unsolicited advice—is a small withdrawal.

The problem is, we're terrible accountants. We rarely stop to process the withdrawals.

Your alarm goes off. Your partner mentions they forgot the milk (again). *Withdrawal.* Your kid refuses to put on their shoes. *Withdrawal.* Your boss sends a "quick question" e-mail right at the end of the day when you're meant to sign off. *Withdrawal.*

You tell yourself it's no big deal. You push through. But you're not actually letting it go; you're just accumulating emotional debt. And that debt accrues interest in the form of resentment, impatience, and disconnection.

Then, one day, your partner forgets the milk *again*, and you don't just get annoyed—you explode. You're not reacting to the milk. You're reacting to the milk *plus the interest on 100 other unprocessed withdrawals.* Your account is overdrawn, and now you're paying the penalty fees. Time for the Reactive Loop to be triggered in full force.

This invisible debt is bankrupting your most important relationships.

It's turning your partners into adversaries, your children into chores, and your colleagues into obstacles. This chapter is about learning how to balance your emotional books *daily*, so you can operate from a place of surplus instead of scarcity.

The Neurobiology of Relationship Triggers

When you encounter a relational Reactive Loop, you may feel your stomach clench, your chest tighten, or your mood shift instantly—before you've even had a chance to think. Mentally, it can feel like being yanked back into old patterns, reacting faster than reason, as if your past and present are colliding in real time.

Here's what's happening in your brain when someone pushes your buttons:

- **The Amygdala Hijack:** Within about 50 milliseconds of seeing that person's face or hearing their voice, your amygdala has already made a snap judgment based on past experiences, well before your conscious mind has a say.

- **The Mirror Neuron Activation:** Your brain has systems—often called mirror neurons—that help you resonate with others' emotions. When someone is anxious or angry, your nervous system can "catch" their mood, instead of just observing it from a distance.
- **The Attachment System Override:** Relationship conflicts can light up the same neural pathways that formed in your earliest bonds. A partner's withdrawal can unconsciously echo childhood experiences of being left, activating primal fear of abandonment.
- **The Stress Contagion Effect:** Studies show stress is contagious; partners' cortisol levels often rise and fall together. When someone you love walks in the door stressed, your body may mirror their stress response even before words are exchanged.

THE "FIRST FLICKER" RULE

The point of maximum leverage isn't after the explosion; it's at the very first sign of smoke. This is a crucial rule for maintaining peace in your relationships (and other areas of your life as well).

THE RULE:
Don't wait for the inferno; tap when you smell smoke.

It is exponentially easier to interrupt a pattern before it gains emotional momentum. In your relationships, the "smoke" is your earliest physical and mental warning sign that you're being triggered. It's not the yelling match; it's the first flicker of irritation.

What to Look For:

- The subtle tightening in your jaw when your partner uses *that* tone of voice.
- The shallow breath you take when your boss sends a one-word e-mail.
- The first critical thought that pops into your head about what your teenager is wearing.

That is the golden window. When you feel that first flicker, don't ignore it. Pause, take 30 seconds, and tap. By neutralizing the charge at a 2 out of 10, you prevent it from ever escalating to a 10.

The Parent Who Found Her Calm in the Storm

Jen lived through every parent's nightmare. Her daughter's mental health crisis was so severe it required multiple residential treatment programs. As Jen watched her child struggle, she felt helpless, terrified, and constantly on edge.

But unlike most parents in crisis, Jen had discovered a secret weapon: daily emotional resets.

"I turned to Tapping regularly to help process my own emotions and worry," Jen explains. "Instead of letting the stress and fear build up all day, I'd tap whenever I felt overwhelmed."

This wasn't about fixing her daughter or changing the situation. This was about Jen showing up as the parent her daughter needed—calm, present, and supportive—instead of anxious, reactive, and overwhelmed.

"Tapping helped me become more aligned so that I could learn to not say the wrong things to my daughter and to show up in the most supportive way possible."

This was the REWIRED process in real time:

- **Recognize:** She recognized the Reactive Loop of her own fear and overwhelm threatening to take over.
- **Interrupt:** She would physically leave the room and tap to interrupt the emotional spiral before it could dictate her actions.
- **Rewire:** She consistently chose a Rewired Response of calm, presence, and support, which became her new default way of showing up for her daughter.

The result? Not only did their relationship heal, but Jen became a stabilizing force in her daughter's recovery instead of an additional source of stress.

"Things have improved significantly, and EFT, along with therapy, played a large role in that."

Jen's story proves that even in the most stressful relationship dynamics, you have the power to change the entire emotional climate by managing your own nervous system first.

What's Your Relationship Reactive Loop?

Remember the movie *Groundhog Day*? Bill Murray's character lives the same day over and over until he learns to respond differently. Most of us are stuck in our own Groundhog Day with our relationships—same triggers, same fights, same routines, same outcomes, wondering why nothing ever changes.

Every relationship has a recurring Reactive Loop. What's yours?

- **The "You Always/You Never" Loop:** (e.g., "You always leave your socks on the floor." "You never listen to me.")
- **The Mind-Reading Loop:** (e.g., "I shouldn't have to ask, you should just know.")
- **The "Fine, I'll Do It Myself" Loop:** (The cycle of resentment and martyrdom.)
- **The Unsolicited Advice Loop:** (One person offers "helpful" solutions, the other feels criticized.)
- **The Pursue/Withdraw Loop:** (One person pushes for connection, the other pulls away.)

NAME YOUR LOOP

Be brutally honest:

- Which loop from the list feels most familiar?
- How long have you been running this pattern? Years? Decades?
- What's your role in keeping this loop alive?
- What are you getting out of staying in this pattern? (Even negative patterns serve us somehow).
- What scares you about breaking it?

Here's why this matters: **These Reactive Loops are the biggest drain on your love and connection.** They are black holes for emotional energy. Rewiring your reaction to these specific glitches is the highest-leverage thing you can do to change the entire dynamic.

The secret isn't changing the other person or waiting for different circumstances. It's learning to respond differently to the same old patterns, in a way that actually serves you and the ones you love.

The Science of Staying Calm Around People

When you're frustrated with someone, your nervous system is essentially saying: "This person/situation is a threat. Deploy defense mechanisms."

Your body floods with stress hormones. Your brain shifts into fight-or-flight mode. Your capacity for patience, empathy, and creative problem-solving goes offline.

This is why you can't "just stay calm" through sheer willpower alone. That's just a fruitless effort to try to override a biological response with good intentions. Kind of like trying to stop being hungry by thinking, "It's all good, I don't need to eat!"

This is why Tapping is so powerful when people are driving you crazy.

When you tap while thinking about the frustrating person or dynamic, several things happen:

- **Cortisol drops:** Your stress hormones decrease, taking your nervous system out of threat mode.
- **Heart rate regulates:** Instead of being revved up for battle, your cardiovascular system returns to baseline.
- **Prefrontal cortex comes online:** The thinking, reasoning, and empathetic part of your brain becomes accessible again.
- **Perspective shifts:** You stop seeing the person as a threat and start seeing them as a human with their own struggles.

You move from a state of threat to a state of safety, which is the foundation for a quieter mind and a body at peace.

This isn't positive thinking. This is biochemical change that makes calm responses truly possible.

Your Daily Relationship Weather Report

Most of us check the weather before leaving the house. We dress accordingly. We bring umbrellas for rain and sunglasses for sun.

But we never check our internal emotional weather before interacting with people. We just hope for the best and wonder why we get drenched in someone else's bad mood or struck by conflict lightning when we weren't expecting a storm.

What if you started each day with an emotional weather check?

"How am I feeling about my partner today? Storm clouds building or mostly sunny?"

"What's my patience level with my kids? Running low or fully stocked?"

"How's my tolerance for my co-worker's habits? Need an umbrella or good to go?"

Then, like checking weather, you could prepare accordingly. Feeling stormy? Do some Tapping before breakfast. Running low on patience? Reset in the car before walking into the house. Anticipating difficult conversations? Preemptively tap to access your calm inner wisdom.

The Unilateral Peace Treaty

Here is the most radical and empowering truth in this entire book: **You only need one person to change any dynamic or pattern in your life that you are fed up with—and that person is you.** And that includes any relationship dynamic that isn't working for you anymore.

We're taught that relationships are a fifty-fifty proposition. That change requires both people to be on board. That's a myth that keeps us stuck. We can spend our whole lives waiting for someone else to change, while our frustration festers and our relationship erodes.

Tapping allows you to sign a unilateral peace treaty with yourself. Because the truth is, when you stop showing up to the battlefield, the other person has no one to fight.

- When Donna stopped being defensive (**Interrupting her Loop**), her husband's attacks had no target.
- When Jen showed up calm (**a Rewired Response**), her daughter's panic had space to breathe.
- When you stop radiating resentment (**your old Reactive Loop**), your family stops walking on eggshells.

This is about changing the energetic dance between you and that person. You don't need their permission. You don't need their cooperation or even their awareness.

You just need to show up to your Choice Point and choose to Interrupt your *own* pattern.

When you change your steps, the dance itself must change. That is how you reclaim your power and your peace.

The Expectation Trap

Here's where many people stumble: They start Tapping on their reactions, secretly hoping it will make the other person change. They're being the "bigger person" as a manipulation tactic. And when the other person doesn't transform on cue? Resentment floods back in, often worse than before.

Let me be crystal clear: **This is about changing yourself because you don't want to be triggered anymore. Period.**

If you're tapping while thinking, "Once I'm calmer, they'll finally see how wrong they are," you're still in the old Reactive Loop. You're still making them responsible for your peace.

True rewiring means releasing your own reactions because you want to show up as your most grounded self. It means breaking patterns because you are tired of the dance and you are choosing a new way forward.

If they change in response, beautiful. If they don't, you're still free of what's been holding you back.

Clarity Through Calm: Making Choices from Your Deepest Truth

If there's one bottom-line truth about Tapping and relationships (really Tapping and anything in your life), it's this: **Tapping helps calm your stress so you can see with new clarity.** And that clarity is powerful.

When you're triggered, your vision narrows. All you can see is the offense, the pattern, the frustration. Your nervous system is screaming "THREAT!" and flooding you with stress hormones that make nuanced thinking impossible. You're unable to access the wise, compassionate part of your brain.

But when you tap away that activation, something remarkable happens. The fog lifts. And what you see might surprise you.

Sometimes, clarity helps you see your partner in a new light, with more compassion, curiosity, and patience. It might help you see your teenager's defiance as their clumsy attempt at independence, or your parent's criticism as their misguided way of showing love.

Clarity can open space for healing and reconnection.

And other times, clarity reveals harder truths, like:

- You've been enabling a dynamic that hurts you
- You've been accepting treatment you don't deserve
- A relationship has run its course and it's time to walk away
- It's time to set a boundary you've been avoiding
- You need to have a difficult conversation

This is why some people unconsciously resist tapping on relationships. Part of them knows that once the emotional charge clears, they'll have to face what's really there. And then they'll have to make choices.

Relationships aren't simple formulas. We all enter them carrying invisible luggage, past wounds, unconscious assumptions, and old protective patterns. And when those get triggered, it's easy to fall into knee-jerk reactions that only reinforce pain.

But when you use Tapping to release those triggers (to calm the stress response in your body), you stop reacting out of old programming. You start *responding* from a place of inner alignment.

And here's the gift of that: Choices made from clarity rather than reactivity are choices you can stand behind. Whether that path leads to deeper connection or necessary separation, it's a path guided by calm awareness and your deepest truth, rather than chaos and confusion.

You don't have to figure it all out right now. Just start with your nervous system. Calm the noise. And trust that clarity will follow.

How to Have Difficult Conversations

One of the most practical applications of Tapping is preparing for and navigating difficult conversations with the people in our lives, whether that's a partner, a parent, a friend, a co-worker, or anyone else in your life.

Tapping helps us find our center and stay centered through conflict. When we go into a tricky conversation feeling imbalanced, it's so easy to get thrown off kilter, and fast. But when we use Tapping to bring calm to our entire systems, we create that strong foundation to hold us centered even when the stress builds or the conversation goes in a direction we didn't expect.

Here's how to use Tapping strategically for difficult conversations:

Before the Conversation: There are a few different ways you can use Tapping to get centered and clear before a difficult conversation.

- Tap on your specific fears about the conversation. "Even though I'm afraid they'll get defensive when I bring up the money issue . . ." This pre-emptive Tapping helps you show up grounded instead of braced for battle.
- Tap while asking yourself: "What does this person need to hear? What do I need to express? What's the outcome that serves everyone?" to help find clarity on what you want to get out of the conversation.
- Tap while you imagine the conversation and rehearse what you want to say. This will help you show up the way you want to show up and feel calmly prepared to assert yourself with confidence.

In-the-Moment, 2-Minute Reset: If things get heated, ask for a pause. Excuse yourself to the bathroom and do a quick round of Tapping. Even 2 to 3 minutes can shift you from a reactive state to a calmer, responsive state. "Even though this conversation is getting heated and I want to lash out . . ."

The Follow-Up Tap: After difficult conversations, we often replay them obsessively and feel caught up in the emotions and energy of the conflict. Tap immediately afterward to process: "Even though that was hard and didn't go how I hoped . . ." This prevents the interaction from calcifying into resentment.

Remember: You're not using Tapping to manipulate the outcome or control their response. You're using Tapping to show up as your clearest, calmest self—the one who can speak truth with love and hold boundaries with grace.

For the Emotional Sponges Among Us

Some of you reading this aren't struggling with explosive reactions. You're struggling with absorption.

You walk into a room and immediately feel everyone's mood. You leave family gatherings feeling like you've been through a washing machine. You're the one everyone dumps on because you're "such a good listener."

Like the other patterns we've explored in this book, being highly sensitive like this is a nervous system response.

If you recognize yourself here, Tapping can help you develop better energetic boundaries. Right now, you're operating like a sponge—soaking up every drop of emotion around you until you're heavy and dripping with other people's feelings. Tapping helps you become more of a mirror—reflecting back understanding and compassion without taking it all on.

This isn't about turning off your empathetic nature. You can still feel deeply and be in tune with others, but you don't have to absorb *their* energy and emotions. It allows you to be a witness to others' emotions without wearing them as your own.

Try this: Before entering any charged situation, tap while saying:

- "I am responsible only for my own emotional state."
- "I can witness others' emotions without taking them on."
- "Their feelings are valid AND they're not mine to fix."
- "I choose to stay in my own energy field."

You can't control how others respond to you, but you can choose to stay centered, grounded, and clear about where you start and they begin.

The Permission You Didn't Know You Needed

As we close this chapter, I want to give you permission for something:

You're allowed to take care of your own emotional state before taking care of everyone else's needs.

You're allowed to tap in the bathroom while your family wonders where you went. You're allowed to take two minutes for yourself before responding to that frustrating text. You're allowed to reset your nervous system before walking into a difficult conversation. You're allowed to set boundaries, to remove yourself from situations that drain you, to protect your own energy.

This isn't selfish. This is strategic. A calm nervous system makes better decisions, has more patience, and responds more lovingly than a stressed one. It's the source of all the core benefits this book promises.

You can't give what you don't have. If you're running on frustration fumes, frustration is what you'll offer. But if you're operating from genuine calm, that's what you'll share.

RECLAIMING *Your* FREEDOMS

The pattern we explored in this chapter doesn't just cause discomfort; it actively steals some of your 7 Freedoms. By using Tapping to rewire this pattern, you're not just getting rid of a problem—you're reclaiming your birthright to a full, vibrant life.

Take a moment to reflect: Which of these freedoms would open up the most for you if this pattern no longer had a hold on you?

- The freedom to experience emotions without being overwhelmed.
- The freedom to respond with wisdom instead of reacting from old wounds.
- The freedom to feel calm in situations that used to throw you.
- The freedom to access energy you didn't know you had.
- The freedom to feel at home and peaceful in your body.
- The freedom to trust yourself to handle whatever comes your way.
- The freedom to show up as your real self, not who you've been conditioned to be.

What is the first thing you would do, create, or experience with this newfound freedom?

Your Relationship Revolution Starts Today

Right now, think about the person who frustrates you most consistently. Feel that familiar irritation rising just thinking about them?

That's your cue. That's your nervous system running its old program: "This person = frustration. Deploy annoyance immediately."

But you're at a Choice Point. You can let that frustration build until your next interaction is tainted by accumulated resentment. Or you can interrupt the pattern right now.

The person who drives you crazy isn't going to magically change. But your relationship with them can transform completely when you start tapping on your reactions instead of collecting evidence of their crimes.

Donna saved her marriage by tapping away her daily irritations before they became explosive fights. Jen supported her daughter's healing by processing her own emotions instead of adding them to the crisis.

They both discovered the same transformative truth: When you change your internal state, you change your relationships. When you process your emotions, you stop projecting them onto others. When you calm your system, you stop making knee-jerk reactions that hurt yourself and others.

And a whole new reality opens up before you. A whole new sense of inner calm and empowerment settles in.

Ready to revolutionize your relationships from the inside out?

Let's tap.

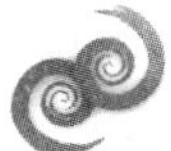

TAPPING SCRIPT: *Staying Centered When Others Push Your Buttons*

Let's start by checking in.

Think about a person or a dynamic that tends to push your buttons.

On a scale of 0 to 10, how stressed do you feel by them? 10 is even the thought of them stresses you out and 0 is feeling calm and at ease.

Take a gentle breath in . . . and out.

Start tapping on the side of your hand. Repeat either in your mind or out loud.

Side of the Hand: Even though they trigger me so quickly,
and I feel drained every time,
I acknowledge how I feel.

Even though I get caught in the same loop again and again,
I'm open to the possibility of a new way forward.

Even though it feels like they take my peace away,
I choose to acknowledge the power I do have.

Eyebrow: I feel the irritation rising
Side of the Eye: My body tenses so fast
Under the Eye: My mind jumps into old stories
Under the Nose: I've been here before
Under the Mouth: The same argument with different words
Collarbone: The same old loop

Under the Arm: All this tension and stress
Top of the Head: I recognize this pattern

Eyebrow: I've been reacting
Side of the Eye: Feeling triggered
Under the Eye: I thought I had to engage
Under the Nose: But this is just the same old loop
Under the Mouth: I now calm my nervous system
Collarbone: I don't have to show up in the same old way
Under the Arm: I don't need to absorb their mood
Top of the Head: I don't need to carry their opinions

Eyebrow: Everyone has their own inner struggles
Side of the Eye: I let go of taking their behavior personally
Under the Eye: I let go of trying to change them
Under the Nose: I focus on grounding my energy . . .
Under the Mouth: and choose to let them be
Collarbone: I'm open to new clarity . . .
Under the Arm: on how to navigate this relationship
Top of the Head: My nervous system is safe to relax

Eyebrow: I now protect my peace
Side of the Eye: My energy is steady and strong
Under the Eye: Feeling more relaxed and safe
Under the Nose: I have nothing to prove
Under the Mouth: I allow myself to just be
Collarbone: I am in my power
Under the Arm: I relax more deeply now
Top of the Head: Feeling a new sense of relief

Gently stop tapping and let your hands rest. Take a deep breath in . . . and let it out slowly.

Bring that person or dynamic to mind again. Where is your sense of inner peace on the 0-to-10 scale now? Notice that your power doesn't come from changing them, but from your ability to stay true to your own calm.

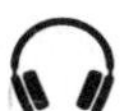
For a guided audio version of this Tapping meditation, visit www.thetappingsolution.com/rewired.

To Remember . . .

The Core Insight: *You cannot change other people, but you can change the dynamic of any relationship by changing your own reaction. You don't need their permission or participation to find clarity and create peace in your own life. When you find your center by interrupting old relationship Reactive Loops and regulating your nervous system, you open up new pathways ahead that allow you to set boundaries, have difficult conversations, and create change.*

The Practice: *Use the first flicker of irritation as your cue to tap, before the emotion gains momentum. Your practice is to take responsibility for your own emotional state by tapping on your triggers* in the moment. *This is an act of self-empowerment that stops you from giving your peace away to someone else's behavior.*

CHAPTER 17

When Money Makes You Panic

Calming Stress Around Finances

There's one thing that touches every single aspect of your life, yet most of us would rather have a root canal than look at it honestly.

It determines where you live and how you sleep at night. It influences who you date and whether you stay together. It affects what you eat, how you move through the world, which dreams you pursue and which you abandon. It even shapes how you see yourself—worthy or wanting, capable or condemned to struggle.

Money.

Just reading that word probably changed something in your body. Maybe your shoulders tensed. Maybe your breathing shifted. Maybe you felt a familiar flutter of anxiety or a wave of exhaustion.

This single word triggers more Reactive Loops than almost any other. Just seeing your bank balance can launch a dozen automatic stress responses.

If that's the case for you, you're not alone. Out of the millions of sessions tracked in our app, financial Tapping sessions consistently show the highest starting stress levels. People rate their money stress higher than their anxiety about health, relationships, or any other topic we cover.

Think about that for a moment. The thing that's supposed to be just a "medium of exchange"—just numbers on a screen or paper in your wallet—triggers more nervous system activation than almost any other life challenge.

Why?

Because money has become the modern language of survival itself.

Your Bank Account Is Not a Bear (But Your Brain Doesn't Know That)

Let's be honest: Nothing hijacks your nervous system quite like money.

And here's why money triggers us like nothing else: To your primitive brain, money equals survival.

More than any other modern stressor, money plugs directly into your ancient survival wiring. To your nervous system, a dwindling bank account isn't just a logistical problem; it's the modern equivalent of a failed hunt or a barren field. It screams, "DANGER! Not enough resources. Starvation imminent. Shelter compromised."

No money = no food = death

No money = no shelter = death

No money = cast out from the tribe = death

This is why you can be a calm, rational person in every other area of your life, but the moment you open your banking app, your heart starts pounding and your breathing gets shallow. It's why financial stress is a leading cause of divorce—it's not just about numbers; it's about a fundamental sense of safety in the world being constantly threatened

And it's also why "just budget better" or "think abundant thoughts" feels about as helpful as someone telling you to "just relax" while you're being chased by a bear.

Your nervous system is in full survival mode. And until you address that, all the financial advice in the world won't stick.

The cruel irony is that the more your nervous system freaks out about money, the less capable you become of making sound financial decisions. Fear shuts down the part of your brain that could help you find solutions.

Many of us have been living with that low-grade (or high-grade) survival alarm blaring on our entire lives, running a Reactive Loop so familiar we've accepted it as "just the way things are."

But it doesn't have to be. We can rewire this pattern.

The Inheritance Nobody Wants

Your relationship with money was programmed before you could even count. It was coded into your nervous system through overheard whispers, tense family dinners, and the things left unsaid. For Heidi, that programming was a legacy of scarcity and fear.

Heidi grew up in Denmark with a father who turned the family motto into "We can't afford that." No sports. No activities. No extras. He poured every penny into retirement savings, only to die young before he could enjoy any of it.

The message was clear: Money is scarce. Life is about deprivation. You'll never have enough. This was Heidi's inherited Reactive Loop: a pattern of scarcity thinking passed down like a family heirloom.

Decades later, when the pandemic shut down her husband's tourism business in Greece, those old programs came roaring back. At her age, with her background, who would hire her? Her friends even echoed what her own inner critic was saying: "You're too old. Nobody's hiring. Remote work is for young people."

But Heidi hit a Choice Point. She could let her father's voice run her life, or she could Interrupt the pattern.

She started tapping. On the fear of not getting a job. On the belief that she had nothing to offer. On the echoing belief of "we can't afford that" that had haunted her for 40 years.

What happened next is a testament to the power of rewiring. As her nervous system calmed, something shifted. The fog of fear lifted enough for her to see clearly: She had skills. She had value. She had options.

She started applying for jobs and, to her own surprise, got hired. Then got promoted. She quickly became a star employee.

For the first time, Heidi felt proud of her ability to contribute financially. She had interrupted a lifelong Reactive Loop and installed a new reality—one of capability and abundance. She wasn't just earning money; she was earning a new sense of self.

When Your Financial Thermostat Keeps You Stuck

My brother, Alex, has a powerful story about how our childhood shaped his relationship with money. He often shares it in our financial programs, because it perfectly illustrates how early experiences create the financial patterns that run our lives as adults.

"When I was eleven years old," Alex began, "my dad lost his job. He'd been laid off by a company he'd worked for since we moved from Argentina to Connecticut when I was four. My parents had brought our family of five to the US with big dreams and few belongings.

"I don't remember my dad telling me he lost his job. What I do remember is going out with him a few weeks later, delivering phone books to earn extra cash. For those of you old enough to remember phone books, those massive directories that got delivered once a year, you know what I'm talking about.

"I can still remember laughing as we drove around neighborhoods, me hanging out the window dropping off phone books. But I also remember the fear that crept in after about a week. What was next? Would we be okay?

"This experience planted deep seeds of patterns of financial scarcity that would run my life for decades."

Alex's story continues with a pattern that might sound familiar to many of you:

"My financial set point, programmed by those childhood experiences, drove me to repeat my father's patterns almost exactly. In college, I started attending real-estate investing seminars. I thought, 'People make money in real estate. If I learn the system, I'll succeed too.'

"Over five years, working with my father and Nick, we flipped over one hundred houses. Sounds successful, right? Not exactly. We were always 'kind of doing well, but not really'—the same pattern my dad had run. Some houses made money; many lost money. We made decision after decision from our financial setpoint."

The 2007 crash hit us hard. As Alex described it: "We owned thirty vacant properties with over a million dollars in personal debt and virtually no cash. Credit cards maxed. Credit lines exhausted. The absolute worst-case scenario had materialized. I felt like a complete failure."

If you've ever been in debt, or if you're in debt right now, you're probably feeling the pain we went through during that time.

And at this lowest of low points, that's when Alex turned to Tapping.

"That's when my life began to shift radically. All the patterns that I was running, all the limiting beliefs and negative emotions that were holding me back, I was able to shift because of Tapping. Tapping helped me to process what I was going through and to understand that failure was a part of the process. Then I used it to get motivated again to build up my belief, to overcome limiting beliefs about what I believed was possible and to keep me going day to day. And man, has my life changed since that time."

Today, Alex lives a life that was beyond his wildest dreams, far from the 11-year-old who laid in his bed staring at the ceiling, wondering what would happen next.

As he put it: "I'm incredibly lucky to say I share a prosperous life with a wife I love and three amazing kids. Yes, there's the house with the pool and all that. But more importantly, there's freedom. I don't stress about money the way I used to. I work because I love helping people, not because I'm running from scarcity."

WHAT BELIEFS DO YOU HOLD ABOUT MONEY?

- ❑ "There's not enough for everyone."
- ❑ "Money isn't spiritual."
- ❑ "Money is hard to come by."
- ❑ "No pain, no gain."
- ❑ "I'm bad with money."
- ❑ "You have to fight for every penny."
- ❑ "I don't deserve wealth."
- ❑ "We can't afford that."
- ❑ "Money changes people."
- ❑ "Wanting money is selfish."
- ❑ "Rich people are greedy/selfish/bad."
- ❑ "People like us don't get rich."
- ❑ "You have to work hard for money."
- ❑ "More money, more problems."
- ❑ "If I make more, I'll just lose it."

THE SPECIFICITY SOLUTION: TAPPING ON THE LEAF, NOT THE FOREST

Once you've identified your general money pattern, the key to rewiring it is to get granular. "Financial stress" is the whole forest—it's too big and vague to tap on effectively. To get results, you must focus on a single leaf. This is the **Specificity Solution**.

THE RULE:
Don't tap on the forest; tap on the leaf.

Your nervous system needs a clear target. Instead of tapping on "I'm stressed about money" (the forest), get specific. Tap on:

- "This knot in my stomach when I see my credit card bill" (the leaf).
- "The memory of my mother worrying about bills at the kitchen table" (the leaf).
- "This feeling of panic when I think about asking for a raise" (the leaf).

If you ever feel like Tapping isn't working on a big issue like money, the answer is almost always to get more specific. Find the one small piece of the problem you can feel *right now*, and start there.

Common Money Patterns That Run Our Lives

I've noticed we all run variations of similar Reactive Loops about money. Here are some common examples:

- **The Scarcity Scanner:** Your brain is constantly calculating what you don't have. Even when bills are paid, you're worried about next month. Even with money in savings, you see only what might go wrong. You live in future lack while surrounded by present abundance.
- **The Guilt Spender:** Every purchase comes with a side of shame. You buy something you need and immediately feel guilty. You treat yourself and instantly regret it. Money becomes associated with moral failure.

- **The Avoider:** You can't look at the numbers. Bills go unopened. Accounts go unchecked. You'd rather live in fearful mystery than face financial reality. What you don't know can't hurt you—except it's hurting you constantly.
- **The Feast-or-Famine Cycler:** Money comes in, you feel temporarily safe, maybe even splurge. Then panic sets in and you clamp down hard. Your relationship with money swings between extremes, never finding middle ground.
- **The Perpetual Underearner:** You consistently charge less than you're worth, accept less than you deserve, or sabotage opportunities for more. Some part of you believes you're not allowed to have financial ease.

Which pattern sounds familiar? Maybe several?

Notice how each one is just your nervous system trying to keep you safe from the "threat" of financial instability. Even the patterns that keep you broke (especially those) are protection mechanisms gone haywire.

These are all variations of Reactive Loops, those automatic stress responses to money that fire without your conscious permission.

The Lemon Ice Cream Panic

Sometimes our money patterns reveal themselves in the smallest moments.

Kerstin was 10 years old when her aunt's wealthy friend Gloria handed her an elegant purse full of money to buy ice cream for everyone. Standing at the counter, holding that expensive purse, Kerstin froze.

The weight of that money—money that wasn't hers, money she might lose or miscount—overwhelmed her. In her panic, she ordered lemon ice cream for everyone. Not because anyone wanted lemon. Because her nervous system was so activated she couldn't think clearly enough to ask for preferences.

"I formed my belief right there," Kerstin realized decades later while tapping. "I cannot handle large amounts of money."

One moment. One stressed child. One lifelong pattern of playing small with money.

Why Money Might Be Your Most Important Pattern to Address

As I've mentioned before, your money patterns affect everything else we've covered in this book.

Can't relax? Hard to feel safe when you're worried about rent.

Mind racing? Money fears feed the 3 A.M. worry committee.

Feeling numb? Sometimes we shut down because feeling our financial reality is too scary. Relationships strained? Money stress is one of the top causes of divorce.

This isn't about becoming rich or manifesting millions (though if that happens, fantastic). This is about breaking the survival-mode patterns that keep you in perpetual financial fight-or-flight.

Because here's what I know: You can't build your greatest life from a state of financial panic. You can't access creativity, intuition, or joy when your nervous system thinks you're one bill away from death.

YOUR MONEY ORIGIN STORY

Take a moment to trace back:

- What's your earliest money memory?
- What phrases about money did you hear growing up?
- What did you learn about money without anyone explicitly teaching you?
- When did money first feel scary, scarce, or significant?

Write down what comes up. Often our entire financial operating system was installed before we were old enough to question it.

From Financial Panic to Financial Peace

Jennifer knew the spiral well. Look at bank account. Feel overwhelm. Start pacing. Cue the critical voice: "There's not enough. It's running out. It always runs out."

She'd been here before. Divorce. Losing her farm. Starting over with nothing. The pattern was so familiar, she could predict every beat.

But this time, she caught herself mid-spiral. "Wait a minute! I do not want to panic anymore when I look at my bank accounts!"

Instead of letting the familiar panic run its course, she went back to basics. She tapped. Not on making more money appear, but on her response to what was there.

"Even though I still don't know where my money is going to come from," she wrote, "I can at least control how I am going to respond and react to my situation."

Same bank balance. Same bills. Completely different nervous system state.

And from that calmer state? Options become visible. Solutions appear. Actions feel possible.

When Your Brain Can Finally Think: The Solution Space

Alex shares a powerful insight from his financial journey: "Here's what nobody tells you about financial problems—they're rarely solved by the same brain that's panicking about them."

When you start Tapping, something fascinating happens.

It's not that money magically appears in your bank account. It's that your brain starts working at full force again. Solutions that had been invisible suddenly become obvious. This is the paradox of financial stress: The more desperately you need solutions, the less capable your stressed brain becomes of finding them. It's like trying to do complex math while someone screams, "HURRY!" in your ear.

When you're in financial panic, your brain simply cannot access:

- Creative problem-solving abilities
- Memory of past successes
- Ability to see patterns and connections
- Confidence to reach out for help
- Energy to take consistent action
- Clarity to prioritize effectively

But when you calm your nervous system through Tapping, all these resources come back online. You don't become a different person; you become yourself, fully resourced.

Here's how this typically unfolds:

Stage 1: The Fog Lifts

Your nervous system calms down. The mental static clears. You can actually think in complete sentences instead of panicked fragments.

Stage 2: Reality Becomes Manageable

You see your actual situation—not the catastrophized version your amygdala was projecting. Yes, there are challenges. But you also can find your way through.

Stage 3: Resources Become Visible

Skills you forgot you had resurface. People who could help come to mind. Options you couldn't see through the panic fog start appearing.

Stage 4: Action Feels Possible

Instead of freezing or flailing, you can take one clear step. Then another. Movement replaces paralysis.

Whatever financial challenge you're facing, some part of you already knows the next step. It's just hard to hear that wisdom when your survival alarm is blaring.

The solutions you need are closer than you think. They're one calm breath, one Tapping session, one nervous system reset away.

The Ripple Effect of Financial Peace

When you heal your money patterns, everything else shifts:

The mom who stopped passing money panic to her kids, breaking a generational chain of scarcity

The entrepreneur who finally charged what they were worth and watched their business transform

The couple who stopped fighting about money because they stopped bringing panic to the conversation

You're Allowed to Feel Good About Money

Right now, as you read this, you're likely carrying decades of financial programming that isn't even yours. Inherited fears. Absorbed limitations. Beliefs installed before you could count.

But here's what's also true: Every one of those patterns can be updated. Not through winning the lottery or landing the perfect job. Through the simple act of calming your nervous system around money.

Heidi did it after 40 years of scarcity programming.

Jennifer did it while facing genuine financial uncertainty.

Kerstin did it by finally understanding why she panicked around money.

They didn't change their bank accounts first. They changed their nervous system's response to money. And from that calmer state, everything became possible.

Money will always be part of life. It will always matter. But it doesn't have to trigger your deepest survival fears every time you encounter it.

Let me give you permission for something radical:

You're allowed to have more than enough.
You're allowed to feel safe with money.
You're allowed to spend without guilt.
You're allowed to save without fear.
You're allowed to earn abundantly.
You're allowed to receive easily.
You're allowed to be bad at math and good with money.
You're allowed to make mistakes and recover.
You're allowed to want more than survival.
You're allowed to thrive.

Your bank account is not a measure of your worth. Your income is not a reflection of your goodness. Your financial struggles are not proof of failure.

These feel radical because we've been taught the opposite. We've been trained to earn our existence, to prove our worth through productivity, to apologize for wanting more than scraps.

These permissions are about healing the Great Forgetting around money. We've forgotten that wanting financial ease isn't greedy. We've forgotten that money can flow without struggle. We've forgotten that our worth exists independent of our net worth.

This isn't about positive thinking your way to wealth. It's about interrupting negative patterns to find your way to peace. And from peace, anything becomes possible.

Ready to calm your financial nervous system?

Let's tap.

RECLAIMING *Your* FREEDOMS

The pattern we explored in this chapter doesn't just cause discomfort; it actively steals some of your 7 Freedoms. By using Tapping to rewire this pattern, you're not just getting rid of a problem—you're reclaiming your birthright to a full, vibrant life.

Take a moment to reflect: Which of these freedoms would open up the most for you if this pattern no longer had a hold on you?

- The freedom to experience emotions without being overwhelmed.
- The freedom to respond with wisdom instead of reacting from old wounds.
- The freedom to feel calm in situations that used to throw you.
- The freedom to access energy you didn't know you had.
- The freedom to feel at home and peaceful in your body.
- The freedom to trust yourself to handle whatever comes your way.
- The freedom to show up as your real self, not who you've been conditioned to be.

What is the first thing you would do, create, or experience with this newfound freedom?

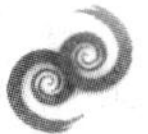

TAPPING SCRIPT:
From Financial Panic to Financial Peace

Let's start by checking in with your financial stress.

Think about your money situation—bills, savings, income, whatever feels most present. On a scale of 0 to 10, how much stress do you feel? 10 being a sense of panic, and 0 being completely at ease.

Take a gentle breath in . . . and out.

Start tapping on the side of your hand. Repeat either in your mind or out loud.

Side of the Hand: Even though money brings up so much stress for me,
I acknowledge these feelings.

Even though thinking about money makes my body tense up,
and I can feel that old panic rising,
I'm open to a new way of relating to money.

Even though I'm carrying old fears about money,
I choose to be gentle with myself as I explore this.

Eyebrow: All this financial stress
Side of the Eye: It lives in my body
Under the Eye: This tightness when I think about money
Under the Nose: These old patterns of panic
Under the Mouth: All these beliefs about money
Collarbone: Money has felt so stressful for so long
Under the Arm: It touches everything in my life . . .
Top of the Head: and I'm tired of being worried

Eyebrow: What if I could feel differently?
Side of the Eye: I'm ready to transform my relationship with money
Under the Eye: I'm not defined by my struggles
Under the Nose: I release any shame from past experiences
Under the Mouth: I was doing the best with what I knew
Collarbone: I acknowledge my growth
Under the Arm: I've already learned so much . . .
Top of the Head: and I'm open to growing in new ways

Eyebrow: I can update my money patterns
Side of the Eye: I can breathe when I think about money
Under the Eye: My body can relax around finances . . .
Under the Nose: so my creativity can come back online
Under the Mouth: I open to options that I couldn't see before
Collarbone: I am capable of finding solutions
Under the Arm: I'm learning to trust myself with money . . .
Top of the Head: and feel hope for the future

Eyebrow:	My confidence is growing stronger
Side of the Eye:	Taking my power back
Under the Eye:	I am shaping my financial future . . .
Under the Nose:	one step at at time
Under the Mouth:	It's safe to relax into this knowledge . . .
Collarbone:	that I am finding my way
Under the Arm:	Allowing my body to relax more deeply
Top of the Head:	Feeling more hope and ease

Gently stop tapping and let your hands rest. Take a deep breath in . . . and let it out slowly.

Check back in with your financial stress. Where is it now on that 0-to-10 scale?

Even a small shift is your nervous system learning that money doesn't have to equal panic.

For a guided audio version of this Tapping meditation, visit www.thetappingsolution.com/rewired.

To Remember . . .

The Core Insight: *Financial stress is a primal survival response. Your nervous system treats money scarcity as a life-or-death threat, hijacking your ability to think clearly. The hopeful truth is that you can separate your sense of safety from your bank balance by calming your body's panic response.*

The Practice: *Your practice is to get granular. Stop tapping on the vague forest of "financial stress" and tap on a specific leaf. Tap on "this knot in my stomach when I look at bills" or "the memory of my parents fighting about money." By neutralizing these specific triggers, you calm your nervous system enough so you can think clearly about money, maybe for the first time in years. From that calmer state, solutions become visible, actions feel possible, and peace becomes available.*

CHAPTER 18

When Life Throws You a Curveball

Building Nervous System Resilience

Picture a master surfer, gracefully carving a line across the face of a massive, churning wave.

No one looks at that surfer and thinks, "Wow, look how brilliantly she is controlling the ocean." The idea is absurd. Her mastery has nothing to do with controlling the raw, unpredictable power of the water. Her genius lies in her ability to *ride* whatever wave comes. She doesn't demand that the ocean be predictable; she cultivates the balance, flexibility, and courage to partner with its power.

And yet most of us spend our lives trying to control the ocean. We build up walls of certainty, and we get angry when an unexpected wave of change crashes over our plans. Our entire sense of safety is tied to the impossible fantasy of making life predictable. This is why a sudden curveball feels so terrifying—it shatters the illusion that we were ever in control in the first place.

Some waves strike out of nowhere: the diagnosis, the disaster, the job loss, the heartbreak. Others are more subtle: the growing discomfort in a relationship, the quiet whisper that you've outgrown your job, the restlessness you can't explain.

In this chapter, we're going to explore both types:

- The kind of change that **happens to you**, forcing you to adapt.
- And the kind of change you **choose to make**, even when you feel uncertain of what is to come.

Both require the same skill: learning to regulate your nervous system so you can respond with clarity, not fear. Ultimately, change asks us to become someone we haven't been before.

This chapter is your surfing lesson. It's time to stop fighting the tides of reality and learn to dance with them. Because your real power isn't in preventing the waves; it's in knowing you can ride them no matter what comes.

The Retirement Dream That Crumbled in Four Hours

September 6, 2017.

Sharone had finally made it. After decades of careful planning, she was living the retirement dream: a paid-off rental house business, a beautiful home completely owned, zero debt except daily expenses. She'd done everything "right." She'd saved diligently, invested wisely, built security brick by brick.

Then Hurricane Irma arrived, the first Category 5 storm to hit her island in recorded history.

"In four short hours, a lifetime's work was demolished, and before I know it, I am being evacuated from the rubble in a helicopter basket."

Picture that for a moment. Waking up financially secure with your future mapped out. Going to bed airlifted from the ruins of everything you'd spent 30 years creating.

All that planning, all that careful execution, gone in just four hours.

"I've lived a deeply spiritual life since I was twenty years old, but I didn't feel prepared for this curveball. While I absolutely knew that this was nothing short of an opportunity to 'walk my talk,' knowing that did not take the trauma out of the situation."

This is the brutal truth about life's curveballs: They don't care about your plans, your preparations, or even your spiritual practices. They arrive without invitation and demand you step up to face it.

THE CHANGE RESISTANCE TEST

Quick–How do you feel about the following statements? Rate each one from 1 to 10 (1 = "totally disagree," 10 = "story of my life"):

____"When my favorite show gets canceled, I'm genuinely upset for weeks"

____"I check the same news websites/apps in the same order every morning"

____"I feel anxious when someone rearranges my workspace or living space"

____"I've been putting off a major life decision for months (or years)"

____"I still use the same passwords I created five years ago"

____"When plans change last minute, I feel stressed even if the new plan is better"

____"I have strong opinions about 'the way things should be done'"

____"I avoid conversations that might lead to conflict or change"

____"I stay in situations that aren't working because at least they're familiar"

____"The phrase 'we need to talk' makes my stomach drop"

Add up your score.

70-100: You're a Change Resistance Champion. You've turned avoiding change into an art form, but life is about to test your masterpiece.

40-69: You're a Selective Change Tolerator. You can handle change when you control the timing and terms. Plot twist: You rarely will.

10-39: You're a Change Flow-er. You roll with life's punches better than most, but even you have limits.

Now no matter how you scored here, there's one thing you need to know: **Life doesn't check your change tolerance level before serving up curveballs.**

The divorce papers arrive whether you "do" relationship drama or not. The medical diagnosis comes whether you're "ready" or not. The job elimination happens whether you handle workplace stress well or not.

Your carefully constructed routines, your comfort zones, your "this is how I like things" preferences–at some point, they're likely to come face to face with the ever-flowing, ever-changing landscape of life.

The Certainty Addiction That's Destroying Your Life

Let's get honest about something: We're all addicted to certainty.

Maybe you fall down the rabbit hole of restaurant reviews, trying to pick a place for lunch with friends, as if there's a perfect choice waiting. Maybe you refresh your weather app six times before leaving the house to meet up with them. Maybe you recheck your texts five times before leaving your car to make sure you got the meetup location right. All that for one lunch.

This isn't careful planning. This is certainty addiction—the desperate belief that if you just gather enough information, you can eliminate uncertainty from your life. It's one of humanity's favorite Familiarity Traps: choosing the "safe" illusion of control over the reality of growth.

But turns out, it doesn't really work that way. **The more you need certainty, the less capable you become of handling uncertainty.**

Think about it. Every time you avoid making a decision because you "need more information," you're actually training your nervous system that uncertainty is dangerous. Every time you postpone action until you can "predict the outcome," you're reinforcing the belief that the unknown is unsafe.

You think you're being careful. But you're actually making yourself more fragile.

Meanwhile, life keeps throwing curveballs, because that's what life does. And each curveball hits harder because you've been building your entire sense of safety on the fantasy that you can control what happens next.

YOUR CERTAINTY CRUTCHES

Be honest with yourself:

- What decisions have you been postponing because you "need more information"?
- How many times today did you check the weather, reread texts, or seek reassurance about plans?
- What's one area where your need for predictability is actually keeping you stuck?

The True Cost of Resisting Reality

Your nervous system has created an elaborate illusion that you're safer when you know what's coming. This is the ultimate Familiarity Trap—confusing predictability with safety.

But think about the most predictable parts of your life right now:

- The job that slowly drains your soul (predictable, but is it safe?)
- The relationship patterns that repeat every few months (familiar, but are they healthy?)
- The financial habits that keep you barely getting by (known quantities, but are they serving you?)
- The health patterns you can predict to the day (routine, but are they sustainable?)

Your nervous system treats these patterns as "safe" because they're known. But predictable misery isn't safety, it's just familiar suffering.

Meanwhile, the changes you're avoiding (the new career, the difficult conversation, the move to a different city, the creative project, the relationship that could be amazing) feel "dangerous" because they're unknown.

Your brain has it exactly backwards: The familiar patterns keeping you stuck are the real danger. The uncertainty you're avoiding is where freedom lives.

And your resistance to change is costing you in major ways:

- **Dreams deferred indefinitely:** How many opportunities have you passed up because you couldn't guarantee the outcome? How many "somedays" have turned into "nevers"?
- **Energy drained by indecision:** All that mental energy spent researching, planning, and avoiding decisions? That's energy not available for actually living your life.
- **Relationships stuck in stagnation:** The conversations you're avoiding, the boundaries you're not setting, the love you're not expressing—all because change feels too risky.
- **Your authentic self, buried under layers of "practical":** Every time you choose familiar over fulfilling, you bury another piece of who you're meant to become.

Without a doubt, there is a cost to all this resistance. And it's not just the opportunities you miss—it's the very texture of your life.

The good news? There's a way out of this trap. But it requires flipping your entire approach to uncertainty. As Tony Robbins puts it, "The quality of your life is in direct proportion to the amount of uncertainty you can comfortably live with."

If nothing changes in your current patterns, where will you be in five years?

The Neuroscience of Why Change Feels Like Death (And Why That's Actually Good News)

There's something that your nervous system doesn't understand about modern life: **Change and uncertainty won't actually kill you.**

But try telling that to your amygdala when your boss says, "We need to talk," or your partner suggests "taking a break."

To your primitive brain, change equals potential danger. This made evolutionary sense when change might mean "new predator in the territory" or "familiar food source disappeared."

But now your brain treats the following situations as equally threatening:

- Moving to a new city (unknown territory = potential death)
- Starting a new relationship (unknown person = potential betrayal)
- Changing careers (unknown challenges = potential starvation)
- Having difficult conversations (unknown outcome = potential abandonment)
- Meeting new people (unknown situation = potential rejection)

Your nervous system processes change as a survival threat, flooding your body with stress hormones designed for immediate physical danger.

This is why unwanted change feels so viscerally terrible. And that reaction isn't just you being too dramatic. It's you having a normal biological response to what your brain perceives as mortal danger.

But here's the good news: Once you understand this is just outdated programming, you can update it.

Proof: The Woman Who Found Peace in the Storm

Barbara's curveball came in an already profoundly time in the world:

"In the very beginning of Covid, my husband was diagnosed with Alzheimer's."

Barbara's retirement dreams—traveling together, growing old gracefully—vanished in a doctor's office, replaced by medical decisions and caregiving.

"My anxiety was overwhelming. I had to make decisions about medication, about whether to enter an Alzheimer's study or not."

Barbara hit her Choice Point in the darkest possible circumstances. She could fall into the familiar pattern of "Why us? Why now? This isn't fair." Or she could interrupt the pattern with something different.

"One day, out of the blue, The Tapping Solution App came across my FB feed. I gave it a shot. It changed my life."

This is the REWIRED process in action:

- **Recognize:** "I'm stuck in anxiety about circumstances I can't control"
- **Interrupt:** Tap instead of spiraling into "what if" thinking
- **Rewire:** "I can handle whatever comes, one day at a time"

Five years later, Barbara's external circumstances haven't magically resolved. Her husband still has Alzheimer's. The future she'd planned is still gone. But her relationship with unavoidable change has been completely Rewired.

"My anxiety is under control most of the time. Now I find myself tapping on things like happiness, gratitude, and peace instead of anxiety."

A woman whose husband has Alzheimer's spends her time tapping on gratitude and peace. Not because she's in denial, but because she discovered something that changed the game forever: **You can't control what happens to you. But you can rewire how you respond to what happens to you.**

And as it turns out, focusing on peace and gratitude makes life a lot more enjoyable than focusing on what could go wrong.

A NEW DEFINITION OF RESILIENCE

We tend to glorify the ability to endure immense pressure without breaking. But this mindset leads to burnout and long-term damage. True strength in the face of life's curveballs looks different. It's time for a new **Definition of Resilience.**

THE RULE:
Resilience is not how much you can endure;
it is how quickly you return to baseline.

Think of a resilient system like a rubber band, not a steel bar. The steel bar is rigid; when it finally breaks, it shatters. The rubber band is flexible; it can be stretched to its limit (the crisis) and then rapidly return to its original shape (your calm baseline).

Stop measuring your progress by the absence of challenges. Start measuring the speed of your recovery. A thought that used to ruin your week now only ruins your afternoon? That is a massive victory in resilience. Tapping is the tool that trains your nervous system to be that flexible, responsive rubber band that can return to baseline frequently and swiftly.

The Two Types of Life Curveballs

Through analyzing thousands of stories like Sharone's, we've identified two distinct types of curveballs that completely derail us:

The Lightning Strike: Hurricane Irma. Cancer diagnosis. Divorce papers. The kind that splits your life into "before" and "after" in a single moment.

The Slow Reveal: The gradual realization that your marriage stopped working years ago. The creeping awareness that your career is sucking your soul. The dawning recognition that your aging parents need more help than you want to admit.

Both are terrifying. Both force you to become someone you've never had to be before. Both require skills you haven't developed yet. Both trigger common Reactive Loops: the "this shouldn't be happening" loop, the "I can't handle this" loop, the "everything is falling apart" loop.

The lightning strike feels like getting hit by a truck: sudden, dramatic, impossible to ignore.

The slow reveal feels like slowly sinking in quicksand: By the time you notice you're stuck, you're already in too deep for easy escape. And you are forced to make a choice—Do I do something about it, or do I keep sinking?

Either way, your nervous system has the same reaction: **"This wasn't supposed to happen. This isn't the plan. I don't know how to handle this. And I don't want to."**

YOUR CURVEBALL INVENTORY

Which type of change are you facing right now?

- ❑ Lightning Strike (sudden, dramatic, undeniable)
- ❑ Slow Reveal (gradual awareness that something needs to change)

When Lightning Strikes a Whole Community

You already know about December 14, 2012, the day the Sandy Hook shooting shattered my hometown of Newtown, when 26 children and six educators were killed.

If you want to talk about a curveball that nobody saw coming, one that split time into "before" and "after" in the most devastating way possible, this was it.

What I haven't shared with you yet is how that tragedy became the ultimate test of everything I'd been teaching about handling life's curveballs.

I'd been teaching Tapping for years by then. Our business was picking up momentum. We had plans, strategies, next steps all mapped out. But when something like that strikes in your hometown in such a devastating way, business plans become instantly irrelevant.

The emotional tension was unlike anything I'd experienced. As a new father myself, the horror hit at a primal level. As someone who taught emotional healing techniques, people looked to me for guidance. But inside? I was a grieving neighbor, terrified parent, and devastated community member just trying to process the unprocessable.

Jessica, Alex, and I faced our biggest Choice Point yet. Stick to our business trajectory or drop everything to help our community.

We founded The Tapping Solution Foundation almost immediately with no business plan, no revenue model. Just a desperate desire to help. We worked with survivors, first responders, teachers, and parents. We'd hold it together during sessions with those who needed support, then break into tears afterward.

Working with Scarlett Lewis days after she lost her six-year-old son, Jesse, taught me something profound: Being a healer doesn't mean you're invulnerable. It means you can use your vulnerability to connect with others' pain.

When Scarlett felt "the first lifting of the weight on my chest" after our Tapping sessions together, I understood we weren't just teaching people a technique. We were handing them a lifeline when life's most devastating curveballs left them drowning in unimaginable pain.

Sometimes purpose doesn't arrive through careful planning. Sometimes it crashes into your life uninvited, demanding you rise to meet it. The question isn't whether you're ready (you're usually not). The question is whether you'll show up anyway.

The Man Who Lost Everything and Found Purpose

Glenn's story shows what becomes possible when you stop fighting inevitable change and start working with it.

Glenn's curveballs came in rapid succession: First his father died, then his brother, then his wife of 34 years. Each loss he could have processed separately, but life doesn't always give you that luxury. Sometimes it compounds grief until you're drowning in change you never asked for.

Those losses were extremely difficult for Glenn. After the final loss of his wife to cancer, he found himself in a painful period of deep, consuming grief and anxiety. At one point, he even thought he was having a heart attack—but later realized it was the intensity of his anxiety building to a breaking point.

At this point, Glenn could have surrendered to bitterness. He could have built walls against any future loss. He could have retreated into safety and predictability.

Instead, Glenn chose something different. He Recognized his pattern of avoiding grief (because it felt too overwhelming), Interrupted it by using Tapping to process it instead of avoiding his feelings, and ultimately Rewired his entire relationship with loss.

After moving through his grief, Glenn came out on the other side and eventually found purpose in his pain. He started a website to inspire others to get outside and lead active lives.

A man who lost everyone chose to help others live fully. This is what becomes possible when you stop resisting change and start collaborating with it.

What would you attempt if you knew you could handle whatever outcome arose?

The Career Change Nobody Planned

Sally's story demonstrates how sometimes life forces the change you've been too scared to make yourself.

"I have been in high-stress roles since I was 18 years old, and now turning 50 this year. From an unstable and dysfunctional upbringing to my first career at 18 years old in the Canadian Armed Forces (Army) for 8 years, 12 years in public health, the last 11 years as a regional office manager."

Thirty-two years of high-stress roles. All that time of pushing through, making it work, staying the course. Then life served up a perfect storm:

"Having a busy family life with my husband raising our two children (ages 18 and 21) with our 21-year-old graduating during COVID, and still experiencing major mental health mood disorders. Taking care of my parents who live across country, my dad passing away in 2023 due to having a cardiac aortic rupture and stroke during COVID, and now taking care of my mom with dementia."

The cherry on top? Job elimination due to company cuts. Everything at once. More than anyone should have to handle.

"I honestly can't think of a time in my life where I wasn't experiencing chronic stress, and two years ago, it all came to a head and shut me down."

Sometimes your nervous system makes the change decision for you. Sometimes "shutdown" is your body's way of saying "this path isn't sustainable anymore."

But here's where Sally's story becomes truly inspiring: Instead of seeing the shutdown as failure, she used it as information.

"I found EFT and I'm well into recovery, and working to build my new career in the mental health space."

The shutdown that felt like an ending became the beginning of work that actually fits her life experience. This is the plot twist hidden in every unwanted change: **Sometimes life forces nudge you toward the change you've always needed.**

And if you're brave enough to listen to those nudges and pursue the new path? Well, the life waiting for you can be truly more beautiful, meaningful, and full of purpose than you ever thought possible.

The Science of Post-Traumatic Growth

Research on "post-traumatic growth" reveals something remarkable: Many people don't just survive major life disruptions, but they emerge stronger, wiser, and more resilient than before.

This growth isn't automatic. It requires what psychologists call "adaptive coping"—the ability to process difficult emotions while remaining open to new possibilities.

This is exactly what Tapping facilitates. When you tap while acknowledging change and uncertainty, several things happen:

- **Cortisol Regulation:** Your stress hormone levels drop, taking your nervous system out of crisis mode and allowing rational thinking to return.
- **Neuroplasticity Activation:** Calmer nervous systems are more adaptable. Your brain becomes more capable of forming new neural pathways and creative solutions.
- **Emotional Processing:** Instead of suppressing difficult feelings about change, you metabolize them fully so they don't get stuck in your system.
- **Perspective Expansion:** With your survival brain quiet, you can access the part of your mind that sees opportunities within challenges, and that can think critically about what to do next.

This is why some people seem to "bounce back" from setbacks while others get stuck. It's not about being naturally resilient—it's about having tools to regulate your nervous system during times of stress, uncertainty, and chance.

As Tina put it, when she discovered the key to handling life's constant curveballs: "Life throws all sorts of challenges, but knowing I can use this amazing method of regulating my body, mind, and spirit each day is a godsend."

Notice she didn't say life stopped throwing challenges. She said she had a reliable way to regulate her nervous system no matter what came.

The Question That Changes the Game

My sister, Jessica, has always been fascinated by transformation stories.

When she had her own podcast, her favorite question to ask guests was: "What is one thing that felt difficult in the moment but ended up becoming the biggest blessing?"

She interviewed everyone from Arianna Huffington to Tim Ferriss to Jim Kwik and other successful entrepreneurs, and the pattern was always the same: The people she admired most had experienced a really difficult moment that, in hindsight, became the catalyst for their greatest growth.

"It's obviously always a lot easier to look back and see how the dots connect," Jessica explains. "But if you can remember in the moment of a crisis that curveballs often turn into our biggest blessings? That can help you navigate the moment with so much more ease."

I know this pattern intimately. When the real estate market crashed in 2008, I watched my carefully built career crumble along with the economy. I'd been working in real estate with my father and brother. Then suddenly, properties weren't selling, deals were falling through, and the stress was crushing.

At the time, it felt like complete failure. I was at a financial rock bottom (a million dollars in debt), feeling lost, and wondering what the hell I was going to do next.

But that economic crash ultimately became my permission slip to pivot toward something that actually aligned with who I was. That "failure" led directly to making our first documentary about Tapping, which led to the books, the app, the Foundation—everything that actually matters in my professional life now. The real estate crash wasn't my ending; it was my beginning. It allowed me to make the choice to change my life, to pursue a new path, and ultimately create the most beautiful life I could imagine for myself.

This isn't about toxic positivity or pretending everything happens for a reason. It's about understanding that some of life's most unwanted interruptions force us toward paths we might never have chosen to step into—paths that end up being exactly where we needed to go.

PAUSE *and* CONSIDER

- Can you think of a past difficulty that ultimately led to growth?
- What qualities did that experience help you develop?
- How might your current challenge be preparing you for something you can't yet see?

Your Choice Point

Right now, you might be thinking about the change you've been avoiding. The conversation you need to have. The decision you've been postponing. The situation that's slowly killing your soul but feels too scary to leave.

Or maybe you're in the middle of an unwanted change right now. Maybe life already threw you your curveball, and you're sitting in the wreckage wondering how to rebuild.

Either way, you're at a Choice Point. You can spend your energy fighting reality (a battle you'll never win), or you can learn to dance with whatever life serves up.

The people in this chapter—Sharone, Barbara, Sally—they all learned to dance. Not because they stopped caring about outcomes, but because they discovered something profound:

Your peace doesn't depend on knowing what's coming. It depends on trusting your ability to handle whatever comes.

That trust isn't something you're born with or without. It's something you can develop through the REWIRED process. By regulating your nervous system during even the hardest of moments, you allow clarity, insight, problem-solving, and perspective to come flowing in.

And that's how you ultimately navigate your way forward one step at a time—even if you can't see the full path just yet.

Every curveball becomes less devastating when you're no longer demanding that life be predictable. Every plot twist becomes an opportunity for growth when you're no longer attached to the story you thought you were living.

If you could talk to yourself five years from now, what would that version of you say about the change you're currently facing and/or resisting?

The Permission You've Been Waiting For

Before we tap, I need to give you permission for something that might feel a little unfamiliar at first:

You're allowed to not know what's going to happen next.

You're allowed to make decisions with incomplete information. You're allowed to change your mind when new information emerges. You're allowed to start things you might not finish and try things that might not work.

You're allowed to be uncertain about your career path, your relationship status, your living situation, your health, your finances, and your future. You're allowed to say "I don't know" without immediately launching into research mode to fix that condition.

You're allowed to live in the question instead of demanding an answer.

This isn't giving up or being irresponsible. This is acknowledging reality: **Life is uncertain. It always has been. It always will be.** And that's not a bug in the system—it's simply a truth of life that makes growth, surprise, and transformation possible.

The uncertainty you've been running from? It's not your enemy. It's the space where all possibilities live. It's where freedom, growth, and authentic aliveness are waiting for you.

RECLAIMING *Your* FREEDOMS

The pattern we explored in this chapter doesn't just cause discomfort; it actively steals some of your 7 Freedoms. By using Tapping to rewire this pattern, you're not just getting rid of a problem–you're reclaiming your birthright to a full, vibrant life.

Take a moment to reflect: Which of these freedoms would open up the most for you if this pattern no longer had a hold on you?

- The freedom to experience emotions without being overwhelmed.
- The freedom to respond with wisdom instead of reacting from old wounds.
- The freedom to feel calm in situations that used to throw you.
- The freedom to access energy you didn't know you had.
- The freedom to feel at home and peaceful in your body.
- The freedom to trust yourself to handle whatever comes your way.
- The freedom to show up as your real self, not who you've been conditioned to be.

What is the first thing you would do, create, or experience with this newfound freedom?

Your New Relationship with Change

When you walk away from this chapter, you won't suddenly love change. You won't become someone who thrives in chaos or seeks out disruption for fun.

But you will have something more valuable: **the knowledge that you can handle whatever comes.**

You'll have a tool that works in helicopter baskets and doctor's offices. In job interviews and difficult conversations. In moments of complete uncertainty and times when everything you thought you knew gets turned upside down.

You'll join the ranks of people who've discovered that the very thing they were most afraid of—change, uncertainty, the unknown—is actually where their power lives.

Ready to stop being who you've always been? Ready to become someone who dances with uncertainty instead of fighting it?

Let's tap.

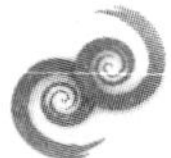

TAPPING SCRIPT: *Finding More Ease Within Change*

Let's check in.

Think about an area of change or uncertainty in your life. On a scale of 0 to 10, how much stress do you feel when you think about it? 10 is feeling very stressed and 0 is feeling completely at ease.

Take a gentle breath in . . . and out.

Start tapping on the side of your hand. Repeat either in your mind or out loud.

Side of the Hand: Even though change can feel unsettling,
and I sometimes worry about what's next,
I acknowledge my feelings.

Even though I've been under a lot of stress,
and I feel all this uncertainty,
I choose to trust my ability to find my way.

Even though life doesn't always go as planned,
I am open to moving forward with greater ease.

Eyebrow: All this uncertainty
Side of the Eye: All this worry
Under the Eye: My racing mind
Under the Nose: My nervous system is on high alert
Under the Mouth: I just want to feel in control
Collarbone: But so much feels out of my control right now
Under the Arm: I acknowledge this stress . . .
Top of the Head: and the toll it has taken on me

Eyebrow: I acknowledge what I can't control . . .
Side of the Eye: and stop fighting against it
Under the Eye: Right now and right here . . .
Under the Nose: I am safe
Under the Mouth: I may not have clarity yet . . .
Collarbone: but I always find my way
Under the Arm: Even in the unknown . . .
Top of the Head: possibilities are waiting

Eyebrow: I don't need to know the whole path . . .
Side of the Eye: I just need to take the next step
Under the Eye: Clarity comes with action
Under the Nose: I trust myself to navigate this
Under the Mouth: I am more resilient than I realize
Collarbone: I am resourceful
Under the Arm: I am creative
Top of the Head: I am strong

Eyebrow: I trust in the path that is unfolding
Side of the Eye: Every experience has taught me . . .
Under the Eye: and prepared me for this new chapter
Under the Nose: I have the tools to handle what comes
Under the Mouth: I relax into this knowledge
Collarbone: It is safe to slow down and support myself
Under the Arm: It is safe to have hope
Top of the Head: I am finding my way through

Gently stop tapping and let your hands rest. Take a deep breath in . . . and let it out slowly.

Tune back in to that situation. What's your number on the 0-to-10 scale now?

The goal isn't to make the uncertainty disappear, but to know you have the inner resources to meet it. When you stop fighting change and start flowing with it, you discover something amazing: You're far more adaptable than you ever imagined.

For a guided audio version of this Tapping meditation, visit www.thetappingsolution.com/rewired.

To Remember . . .

The Core Insight: *Your power isn't in preventing life's unpredictable waves; it's in your ability to ride them with greater ease. Resilience is not measured by how much you can endure, but by how quickly you can regulate your nervous system and rebound to a calm baseline. This is a skill you can develop.*

The Practice: *When change feels overwhelming, your practice is to tap on the feelings of uncertainty. Acknowledge the fear of the unknown. Acknowledge your resistance and worry. By calming your nervous system in the middle of the storm, you gain access to the clarity, creativity, and courage you need to navigate whatever comes your way.*

CHAPTER 19

When You Come Back to Life

Living with Energy, Joy, and Presence

Imagine walking through a museum dedicated to your old life, called "The Museum of Your Former Self." Each exhibit showcases a different version of who you used to be:

The Anxiety Wing displays your 3 A.M. worry sessions, complete with audio loops of catastrophic predictions that never came true. The Perfectionism Gallery features an endless to-do list that somehow never got shorter, no matter how much you accomplished. The People-Pleasing Theater runs a continuous film of you saying yes when you meant no, nodding when you disagreed, apologizing for taking up space.

In my own museum, there's a whole wing dedicated to "Passive Nick"—the guy who thought life just happened *to* him. That exhibit feels like looking at someone who lived their whole life not knowing they could steer their own ship or carve their own path.

As you wander through the halls of your museum, studying the artifacts of your former patterns, something strikes you as profoundly odd: You feel like you're looking at someone else's life.

These behaviors, these reactions, these ways of being that once felt so definitively "you"? They now seem completely foreign and unfamiliar.

Interesting historical relics, but completely irrelevant to how you live now.

This is what recovery actually feels like. Not a dramatic transformation where angels sing and everything turns golden. More like stepping out of a costume you'd been wearing so long you forgot it wasn't your actual skin.

For the last 17 chapters, we've been working to release the patterns that keep us stuck so we can reclaim the 7 Freedoms of a Rewired Life.

So what does it actually feel like when you step out of the prison of your old patterns and into that freedom? It feels, surprisingly, like coming home to yourself.

If you created a museum of your former self, what would be in it? How much of it still feels like "you," versus historical, outdated artifacts?

THE IDENTITY UPDATE PROTOCOL: CLOSING THE LAG

If you feel a strange disconnect looking at that museum of your past, you're experiencing a common phenomenon in transformation: identity lag. Your nervous system has already been rewired, but your conscious story about yourself hasn't caught up yet. To make your changes permanent, you must perform a manual override, a process I call the **Identity Update Protocol**.

THE RULE: Your nervous system state updates faster than your self-perception. You must consciously update your sense of identity to match your new reality.

You may no longer have panic attacks, but you still think of yourself as "an anxious person." This outdated identity acts like a gravitational pull, trying to drag you back into old patterns.

What to Do: Actively install the new identity with Tapping. Use Tapping to anchor in the new belief: "Even though I used to be someone who worried constantly, I am now someone who handles challenges with calm and clarity." You have to consciously give your brain the new script to read from.

The Suspiciously Ordinary Revolution

Sarah woke up at 6:45 A.M. on a Tuesday, just like she had for months. Same alarm. Same bedroom. Same life.

But something was different, even though she couldn't name it immediately.

For the first time in years, she didn't immediately reach for her phone to check for anxiety-inducing news. She didn't mentally rehearse her day while her chest tightened with familiar dread. She didn't negotiate with herself about getting out of bed.

She just . . . got up. Made coffee. Looked out the window at her neighbor's garden and actually saw it—the way morning light caught the tomato plants, how the cat was hunting something in the basil—instead of seeing through it while her mind raced ahead to her 9 A.M. meeting.

Nothing in her external world had changed. Same job, same relationship, same challenges. But it dawned on her that she actually felt like she was living her life instead of surviving it.

This is what nobody tells you about real healing: It doesn't feel like fireworks or movie moments. It feels like finally being able to breathe normally after holding your breath for decades.

The most profound changes often register as the most natural ones. Peace, it turns out, is remarkably . . . livable.

As Leonie discovered: "I use Tapping every day. It really helps me let go of difficulties I'm struggling with and get to sleep . . . and it helps me breathe into joy."

Breathe into joy. What a beautiful way to describe what becomes possible when you're no longer suffocating under the weight of old patterns.

When Your Internal Corporation Gets New Management

For years, you've been running a spectacularly inefficient internal company. Most of your resources were allocated to departments like:

- The Worry Department (working overtime on scenarios that never materialized)
- The Self-Criticism Division (providing 24/7 commentary on your inadequacies)
- The People-Management Office (somehow responsible for controlling other people's emotions)
- The Future Catastrophe Prevention Unit (scanning for threats in grocery stores and e-mail inboxes)

These departments consumed enormous amounts of energy while producing pretty much no useful output. It's like having a factory that runs three shifts a day to manufacture . . . absolutely nothing.

Then one day, the corporate restructuring happens. Not through downsizing or hostile takeover, but through simple reassignment. All that energy gets redirected to departments that actually serve your life:

Curiosity instead of worry.

Creativity instead of criticism.

Connection instead of control.

At first, you might start noticing it in small ways. Having opinions about what you want for dinner again, instead of just eating whatever is easiest because you're too drained to have preferences.

Then, maybe in larger ways: Maybe you start saying no to things that felt obligatory. Or starting to write, paint, or play music again for the first time in 15 years. Or booking a trip abroad that you've been "someday-ing" for a decade.

This isn't about becoming a different person. It's about finally having the bandwidth to be who you actually are underneath all that old programming.

Look, I've been in this field for 20 years now, and I can tell you something with absolute certainty: The amount of energy people waste on internal chaos is staggering. When that energy gets freed up and redirected toward your actual life? That's when everything changes.

Jason puts it perfectly: "Tapping has made an enormous difference in my life. It has allowed me to access levels of healing that I never thought possible. It has been transformational for me, and I am so grateful that I found it when I did."

The Return of Emotional Weather

One of the most surprising discoveries people make is how much their emotional range expands once they stop being dominated by a few overactive patterns.

People who've been emotionally numb for years often describe it something like this:

"I thought healing meant feeling good all the time. Instead, I feel a wide range of emotions, but with more clarity and ease. It doesn't feel 'bad' anymore. I can be genuinely sad about hard events without spiraling depression. I can feel frustrated at something without it contaminating my whole week. I can be happy without bracing for the inevitable crash."

This is what I call emotional freedom: not the absence of difficult feelings, but the presence of choice about how you dance with them.

When your nervous system isn't constantly in protection mode, emotions become like passing weather instead of emergencies. Anger rolls through like a thunderstorm—intense but temporary, clearing the air rather than destroying everything. Sadness falls like necessary rain. Joy arrives like unexpected sunshine.

You develop what researchers call "emotional granularity"—the ability to distinguish between 50 shades of feeling instead of just "good," "bad," and "numb." You can feel the nuances between your feelings, and understand and acknowledge them with greater ease.

This is what amazes me about this process: People discover they're not "naturally" anxious or depressed or angry. They were just running old software that no longer serves their current reality.

Chloe experienced this firsthand: "I had never given meditation a chance before and was skeptical, but I am forever changed for the better."

Forever changed for the better. Let those words truly sink in. Not temporarily improved. Not slightly better. Forever changed.

CHECK-IN

Which of the 7 Freedoms do you feel most connected to right now? Which still feel distant?

1. The ability to experience emotional freedom
2. The ability to respond rather than react
3. The ability to feel calm in situations that used to throw you
4. The ability to access energy you didn't know you had
5. The ability to feel at home in your body
6. The ability to trust yourself to handle whatever comes
7. The ability to show up as your real self

Your New Relationship with Problems (Spoiler: They're Still There)

Perhaps the most practical shift is how you relate to life's inevitable difficulties. Problems don't disappear when you rewire your patterns. Let me be crystal clear about that. But your relationship with them transforms completely.

Before: Problem = Crisis = Overwhelming emergency requiring immediate panic

After: Problem = Information = Situation requiring thoughtful response

This shift is what I've come to think of as "problem resilience"—the ability to face difficulties without being overwhelmed by them. This doesn't mean you don't ever feel stressed or frustrated. It simply means stress and frustration become temporary visitors rather than permanent residents.

And the difference between something ruining your entire day, your week, your month and it just throwing you off for a few moments? This honestly might be the most life-changing aspect of the entire process. When you're not constantly in reactive mode, when you can actually think clearly during challenges, your capacity to navigate life increases exponentially.

The Productivity Paradox (Or: How Doing Less Gets You More)

Something counterintuitive happens when you stop forcing yourself to be productive: You become effortlessly effective.

This isn't about being lazy. It's about working with your nervous system instead of against it. When you're not burning energy on internal resistance, that energy becomes available for focused action.

Antoinette described it beautifully: "I've been having some of the most productive workdays I've had in a long time. I've had random awesome things happen, and I feel this energy within me. Finally, I don't just have the vision of accomplishing great things and freedom in my life; I'm actually working towards it and feeling fantastic."

I've observed something remarkable over the years: A regulated nervous system is an efficient nervous system. When you're not running background programs of worry and self-doubt, your mental processing power increases dramatically. Decision making becomes faster and more intuitive. Creative solutions appear more readily. You can focus deeply without forcing it.

And as Antoinette experienced, that leads to "random awesome things happening" left and right in your life.

Projects you'd been avoiding for years suddenly get completed, not through willpower but through the simple absence of internal friction. Opportunities pop up you weren't expecting. You feel a sense of freedom and possibility that were never there before.

Myra discovered this transformation extended far beyond productivity. For her, Tapping was "A transformational journey, one which has rewarded me richly: mentally, physically, spiritually and financially. . . . With Tapping, all things are possible."

All things are possible. When you stop fighting your own nervous system, when you stop burning energy on internal chaos, you discover capacities you didn't know you had.

Tapping as a Lifestyle: Making This Stick

The secret to maintaining your transformation isn't doing more Tapping; it's weaving Tapping so seamlessly into your daily rhythm that nervous system maintenance becomes as automatic as checking the weather.

I get this question all the time: "How long do I need to keep tapping?" And here's my honest answer: You don't need to tap forever, but you *get* to tap forever. It can become something as normal in your daily routine as brushing your teeth is—not a chore, just hygiene for your nervous system.

The Micro-Moment Method

Instead of waiting for emotional emergencies, practice these miniature interventions:

The Three-Second Reset: Before responding to any trigger—text message, difficult person, stressful news—tap your karate chop point three times while taking a breath. This micro-pause interrupts automatic reactivity and creates space for conscious choice.

Traffic Light Therapy: Use red lights as cues to check in with your body. Tap your collarbone while asking, "What am I carrying that I could release right now?"

Bathroom Break Breakthroughs: Transform necessary bathroom breaks into 30-second emotional check-ins. It's the only place you're guaranteed privacy for a quick reset.

The Threshold Ritual: Tap for 60 seconds every time you cross a threshold—entering your home, starting work, beginning a difficult conversation. This helps you show up fresh instead of carrying residual energy from previous interactions.

Your Cues to Remember

The biggest challenge isn't knowing how to tap, but remembering to do it when old patterns try to reassert themselves.

The Velcro Principle: Attach Tapping to existing habits you never forget. Tap while coffee brews, during commercial breaks, while phones charge, before checking social media.

Follow Your Body's Signals: Train yourself to recognize your unique early warning signs—jaw tension, shoulder tightness, sudden fatigue, racing thoughts. These become your internal notification system to tap before patterns fully activate.

The 2% Rule: Aim to tap on 2 percent of your daily triggers. Not everything, not even most things, just 2 percent. If you experience 50 minor stresses per day, tapping on just one creates momentum for lasting change and endless ripple effects.

Environmental Anchors: Place subtle visual reminders in strategic locations: a small stone on your desk, a bracelet that catches your eye, a plant by your workspace. These anchor the practice in your physical environment.

What Your Life Actually Looks Like Now

Six months from now, if you truly integrate these tools, something new becomes possible:

You wake up and your first thought isn't about everything that could go wrong today. You have opinions about what you want for dinner. You say what you mean without rehearsing it 17 times first. You rest without guilt. You work without constant self-criticism. You love without keeping score.

Problems still exist, but they feel like puzzles to solve rather than evidence that you're doomed. Difficult emotions visit but don't move in permanently. Change becomes interesting rather than terrifying.

You become the person others want to be around, not because you're perfect, but because you're present. Not because you have all the answers, but because you're comfortable with questions.

Like 72-year-old Gary from earlier, who didn't just get rid of back pain with Tapping but whose wife reported also became more patient, calm, and tolerable.

What really gets me excited about this? You stop trying to fix yourself because you finally understand you were never broken. You were just running software that no longer served your current reality.

Carol captured this transformation perfectly: "For anyone considering Tapping, please do it. **It can and does change your life because it changes you.**"

It changes **you**. Not your circumstances. Not your challenges. Not your external world. You. And when you change, everything else shifts in response.

If you fully trusted that this new baseline was permanent, what would you create? What would you dare to dream?

The Permission You've Been Waiting For

You're allowed to be well. You're allowed to feel good. You're allowed to be happy without earning it, calm without justifying it, peaceful without proving you deserve it.

You're allowed to take up space with your joy, your creativity, your fully expressed aliveness. You're allowed to laugh without apologizing, dream without permission, love without conditions, and live without constant self-improvement projects.

You're allowed to let things feel easy.

The old programming that suggested otherwise was just software, not scripture. And now you know how to update the software whenever those obsolete programs try to run.

The museum of your former self is an interesting place to visit, but you don't have to live there anymore. Your new life, this ordinary, livable, remarkably peaceful existence, is waiting.

And you know what? We've been here all along, waiting for you to come back to life.

Welcome home.

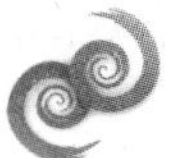

TAPPING SCRIPT: *Expanding Into What's Possible*

Let's start by checking in.

Rate your current stress on the 0-to-10 scale, 10 being overwhelmed and anxious and 0 being hopeful and at ease.

Take a gentle breath in . . . and out.

Start tapping on the side of your hand. Repeat either in your mind or out loud.

Side of the Hand: Even though I've been a certain way for so long, I'm not defined by my past.

Even though I might feel hesitant at times, I choose to trust in the journey that's unfolding.

Even though I still have moments of doubt, my belief in myself is growing stronger.

Eyebrow: My nervous system is updating . . .
Side of the Eye: and my sense of self is catching up
Under the Eye: I'm not my old patterns
Under the Nose: I don't have to fit into old labels
Under the Mouth: I am a wonderful work in progress
Collarbone: I'm becoming more myself each day
Under the Arm: It's safe to keep exploring and growing
Top of the Head: It's safe to expand who I am

Eyebrow: Something is shifting inside of me
Side of the Eye: I can feel new possibilities stirring
Under the Eye: I'm open to new ways of experiencing life
Under the Nose: My emotional range is expanding
Under the Mouth: Feelings can move through me with more ease
Collarbone: I can feel sadness without drowning
Under the Arm: I can feel anger without it taking over
Top of the Head: I can feel joy without fearing it will vanish

Eyebrow: Life is beginning to feel more rich
Side of the Eye: Like spring after a long winter
Under the Eye: Energy beginning to build
Under the Nose: Creativity beginning to flow
Under the Mouth: I'm allowed to take up space
Collarbone: I'm allowed to live without trying to control everything
Under the Arm: I'm allowed to let life feel easier
Top of the Head: I'm allowed to notice what is going well

Eyebrow: I trust what's unfolding
Side of the Eye: My capacity for joy is expanding . . .
Under the Eye: and there's so much more to come
Under the Nose: I'm writing a new story for myself
Under the Mouth: One of vitality and meaning
Collarbone: Of living more authentically
Under the Arm: Feeling excited about the possibilities
Top of the Head: This is just the beginning of something new

Gently stop tapping and let your hands rest. Take a deep breath in . . . and let it out slowly.

Check back in and notice how you feel. What's your current stress level on the 0-to-10 scale?

Like a garden coming back after winter, your aliveness is already there, waiting to bloom in its own perfect timing. Every tap is simply a reminder to your nervous system of what it already knows: You are safe, you are capable, and you are free to be exactly who you are.

For a guided audio version of this Tapping meditation, visit www.thetappingsolution.com/rewired.

To Remember . . .

The Core Insight: *True transformation often feels less like fireworks and more like coming home to yourself. The most important truth you can let sink in is that you were never broken; you were just running outdated software. A sense of peace and ease is possible, and it can become your true baseline.*

The Practice: *Your new practice is to consciously update your identity to match the changes that are taking place deep within you. When an old pattern tries to surface, meet it with Tapping and anchor in your new truths: "I am calm and capable." "I can handle whatever comes my way." "I make empowered choices."*

Afterword

A Rewired Future: The Movement You're Now Part Of

It's 7:23 A.M. on a Wednesday, and I'm drinking coffee in my kitchen when my phone buzzes with an e-mail from Gia that stops me mid-sip:

> *"I've been using Tapping in the classroom for almost 5 years now. The impact it has had on my life, my students' lives, and even my family is incredible. Being able to refocus my students, calm anxieties, and help manage students' emotions has changed the way I teach and the way kids learn when they are under my care. Some of my students have even been using the technique in everyday life outside the classroom. This is the greatest gift as an educator. I know I'm making a difference in many lives because I see evidence within minutes of tapping in the classroom! Children focus better, feel calmer and safer after we tap. I've even noticed they feel more sympathetic towards each other and themselves. I'm so grateful to have this tool as an educator and as a human!"*

I get e-mails like this every day. Thousands of them. Each one a small revolution. Each one proof that what started in my living room with a crick in my neck has become something far bigger than any of us imagined.

When Jessica first read this e-mail, she actually asked me if it was real. And yes, what we shared above was word-for-word, the full message we received from Gia.

My favorite part of that e-mail is this: It's not just about one teacher learning a technique to help her feel more calm. It's about helping the kids she's teaching to feel calmer and safer. It's about an entire classroom of people—adults and kids alike—experiencing the power of Tapping. And the ripple effect that this leads to outside of the classroom.

That's the movement you're now part of. Not just your personal transformation, but the transformation of everyone your nervous system touches.

What Started in My Living Room

Twenty years ago, Tapping was the weird thing I did alone in my apartment when my neck hurt. Today, I've facilitated millions of sessions worldwide through our app alone. But those numbers don't tell the real story.

The real story is in hospitals where nurses are teaching patients to tap before procedures. It's in corporate boardrooms where executives are taking "Tapping breaks" instead of stress-smoking in parking lots.

It's in living rooms like mine, where people discover they don't have to be who they've always been.

But most importantly, it's in the quiet moments when someone chooses to interrupt an old pattern instead of repeating it. When a parent takes three breaths and taps on the side of their hand instead of yelling at their child. When a veteran uses Tapping to sleep through the night for the first time in years. When a retired couple tap together when they feel overwhelmed by the news in the world.

Each of these moments is a small rewiring. Each rewiring creates a ripple. Each ripple becomes part of a wave that's changing how humanity relates to stress, trauma, and emotional pain.

The Accidental Revolution

Here's something that still amazes me: We never set out to start a movement. We just kept sharing something that worked.

When my sister, Jessica, first tried Tapping for her cold, she didn't think, "I'm about to become part of a global revolution in nervous system regulation." She thought, "My brother is probably pranking me again, but I'm desperate enough to try anything."

When we made our first documentary, we weren't planning to reach millions. We were just a couple of regular people with maxed-out credit cards and zero filmmaking experience, hoping maybe someone would benefit from learning about this weird technique.

When we launched our first Tapping World Summit in 2009, we thought maybe 5,000 people would sign up. Over 50,000 registered. Today, that event reaches over 500,000 people annually.

This grew organically because it works. Because when people discover they can tap away their anxiety in a grocery store parking lot, they text their sister about it. When someone sleeps through the night for the first time in years, they mention it to their support group. When a parent finds they can stay calm during their teenager's meltdown, they share it with other parents.

What we're lucky enough to witness now is the viral spread of emotional freedom.

Beyond Individual Healing: The Ripple Effect

What excites me most about where this is heading is that it's not just sparking individual transformation; it's sparking systemic change.

Through The Tapping Solution Foundation, we've brought Tapping to entire communities dealing with collective trauma. After natural disasters. In schools with high stress levels. To veterans' groups struggling with PTSD. To healthcare workers burning out during the pandemic.

The results are consistently remarkable, but what's most striking is how quickly the benefits spread beyond the people we directly work with. When teachers learn to regulate their own nervous systems, their classrooms become calmer. When first responders have tools for processing trauma, they're more present with the people they serve. When parents learn to stay centered during chaos, their children feel safer.

Sometimes the most profound teachers of this ripple effect come in the smallest packages.

Kathleen, an early childhood educator who regularly uses Tapping in her classroom, shared a story that perfectly illustrates how one person's awareness can transform an entire environment.

In Kathleen's class, she had a nonverbal autistic student who seemed to respond to Tapping particularly well. During moments of classroom chaos—when energy was high and focus was scattered—this young boy would quietly approach her and start tapping on his own body to communicate he wanted to tap.

At first, Kathleen assumed he was asking to tap for himself, to regulate his own nervous system. But when she didn't immediately notice his signals, he would gently take her hand and begin tapping on it, making his request impossible to miss.

"I thought he just needed to calm himself down," Kathleen told us. "But then I started noticing a pattern. He wasn't asking to tap when he was dysregulated. He was asking to tap when the classroom was dysregulated."

This child, who couldn't speak, had become the nervous system barometer for an entire room. He could feel the difference between a space full of chaotic energy and one full of calm, focused children. More remarkably, he knew exactly what would shift that energy.

Think about the wisdom in that. A child who processes the world differently than most figured out what many adults miss: Individual regulation creates collective regulation.

This is the future we're building: a future where nervous system regulation isn't seen as individual self-care but as collective care.

Imagine if nervous system regulation was as common as hand washing. If emotional first aid was taught alongside physical first aid. If every workplace had someone trained in helping colleagues process stress before it accumulated into burnout.

This is already happening in pockets around the world. And every one of you who learns to tap, who shares it with someone else, who models what regulated looks like—you're making this future more possible.

You Are the Keystone

In the 1990s, scientists conducted a wild and beautiful experiment. They reintroduced a small number of gray wolves—a species that had been hunted to extinction in the area 70 years earlier—back into Yellowstone National Park. The results were more magical than anyone could have predicted. The wolves changed the behavior of the elk, which allowed the overgrazed willow and aspen trees to recover along the riverbanks.

The return of the trees brought back songbirds. The stronger roots stabilized the riverbanks, which literally changed the course of the rivers, making them meander less and pool more. This created new habitats for beavers. The beaver dams created homes for otters, muskrats, and fish. The wolves are what ecologists call a **keystone species**—a single element that, when present, creates a cascade of positive changes that brings the entire ecosystem back into health and balance.

When you learn to regulate your own nervous system, you become the keystone species in the ecosystem of your life. Your calm changes the behavior of your family. Your regulated presence allows new trust and connection to grow. Your stability changes the emotional flow of the rooms you enter.

The Stories Yet to Be Told

Right now, someone is discovering Tapping for the first time. Maybe they're desperate, having tried everything else. Maybe they're skeptical but curious. Maybe they're in crisis and need something that works faster than traditional approaches.

In a few hours, they'll experience their first shift. Their shoulders will drop. Their breathing will deepen. Their racing thoughts will slow. And they'll have the same reaction you probably had: "Wait . . . what just happened?"

In a few weeks, they'll realize they haven't had a panic attack in days. Or they're sleeping through the night. Or their chronic pain has decreased. Or they're not snapping at their kids.

In a few months, they'll look back and barely recognize the person they used to be. They'll start sharing Tapping with others because they can't help it. Because when you find something that changes your life, keeping it to yourself is impossible.

This story is being written by millions of people right now. Every person who chooses to interrupt their old patterns instead of repeating them. Every tap, one after another.

You're part of this story now. Your transformation matters not just for you, but for everyone your life touches.

What You've Joined

By learning to tap, you've joined something much bigger than a self-help technique. You've become part of a global community of people who've discovered that change is possible, accessible, and simpler than we were taught to believe.

This community includes:

- The single mom who taps in her car before parent-teacher conferences
- The surgeon who does a quick round before difficult operations
- The teenager who teaches Tapping to friends dealing with test anxiety
- The trauma survivor who's become a peer counselor
- The executive who transformed her company's stress culture
- The veteran who helps other vets sleep peacefully
- The teacher who creates calm classrooms through nervous system awareness

What connects all these people isn't demographics or geography; it's the understanding that we don't have to be prisoners of our programming. That nervous systems can be rewired. That suffering isn't permanent. That we all have more resilience and capacity than we've been led to believe.

And let me tell you, this community shows up in the most unexpected places.

Early on, after we released our documentary, we heard a story that still gives me chills to this day. It's always stuck with me! A veteran was walking into Walmart when he got overwhelmed, the familiar panic rising, the crowds too much, the fluorescent lights too bright. Right there in the entrance to the store, he started tapping.

Another vet happened to pass by and recognized what he was doing. As he walked by, without stopping, he simply said, "Keep tapping, it works!" before heading out the doors.

Two strangers. No formal introduction. No lengthy explanation. Just one person recognizing another using the same tool for the same battle. That's the REWIRED movement in action—people who've found something that works, quietly encouraging others to keep going.

Your Role in What Comes Next

The future of this movement isn't determined by conferences or organizations or apps. It's determined by people like you, living from your new wiring, modeling what's possible when someone learns to work with their nervous system instead of against it.

Every time you tap instead of spiral, you're voting for a different future. Every time you stay regulated during stress, you're showing others what's possible. Every time you respond instead of react, you're demonstrating that change isn't just possible; it's practical.

You don't need to become a practitioner or teach workshops (though you certainly can). You don't need to start a foundation or speak on stages. You just need to live as proof that people can change. That old patterns don't have to be permanent. That peace is possible.

The most powerful form of activism is living as an example of what you want to see in the world.

The Invitation

As we close this book, I want to extend three invitations:

First, keep going. Don't let this book become another self-help attempt that fades after initial enthusiasm. Your nervous system is like a garden, and it needs consistent tending. Keep tapping. Keep choosing new responses. Keep proving to yourself that you really have been rewired.

Second, share it. Not because you need to convince anyone, but because this technique works best when it spreads organically through communities of people who care about each other. When someone you love is struggling, offer to tap with them. When a colleague seems stressed, mention what's helped you. When your child is upset, teach them this tool they can use for the rest of their life.

Third, stay connected. Through our app, our community, our events—whatever feels right for you. This isn't about staying dependent on external resources. It's about remaining part of a community that understands what you've experienced and supports who you're becoming.

You've Been Rewired. Now Pass It On.

As I finish writing this book, I'm filled with hope and optimism as I look to the future. Because you know what?

Your story starts now.

You've learned the technique. You've experienced the shifts. You've begun the rewiring process. You understand that your nervous system can be updated, that old patterns don't have to be permanent, that peace is possible.

But most importantly, you've proven to yourself that you don't have to be who you've always been.

Now, go live as proof of what's possible. Go show your children, your friends, your community what it looks like when someone learns to work with their nervous system instead of against it.

Go be the calm presence in chaotic rooms. Go be the person who responds instead of reacts. Go be living evidence that change is possible, accessible, and simpler than most people believe.

The world needs more people who understand that suffering isn't permanent. That patterns can be interrupted. That nervous systems can be rewired.

The world needs you, rewired and living from your new programming.

You've been rewired. Now pass it on.

The future is counting on it.

Your REWIRED Journey Continues Here

You've just learned how to interrupt old patterns and rewire your nervous system for peace, clarity, and resilience.

Now imagine having guided tapping sessions—supporting you every day—right when you need them most.

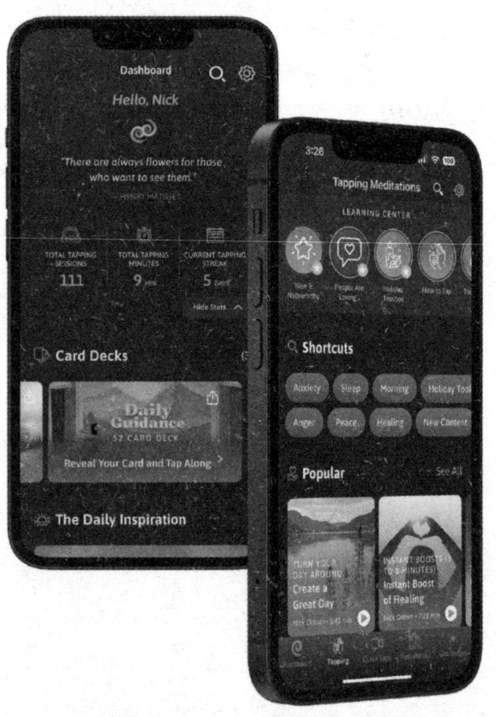

- Guided Tapping for overwhelm, stress, sleep, anxiety, fear, and more
- Sessions that match every chapter of Rewired
- Daily support
- Track your emotional changes in real time

You've already started rewiring.

Let's keep going—tap by tap.

Scan to Unlock Your Free REWIRED Collection

Tap along with sessions created to help you continue your transformation beyond this book.

Scan with your phone's camera to begin instantly.

Appendix A

Tapping Points Reference Guide

The Tapping Points

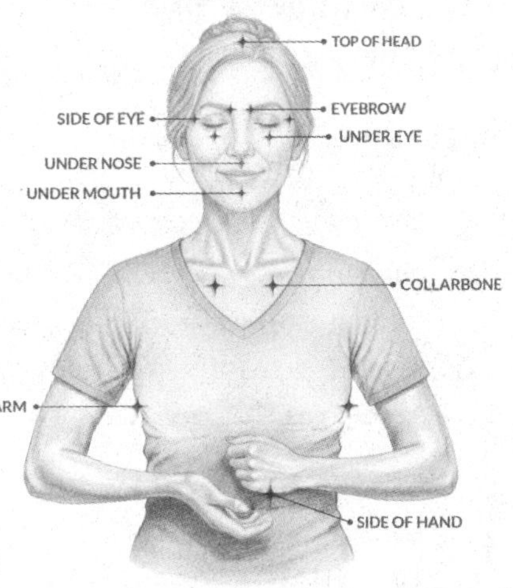

For a video guidance on where and how to tap, visit www.thetappingsolution.com/rewired

1. Side of the Hand (SH)

Location:

The Side of the Hand point is found along the fleshy, narrow side of the hand on the side of the pinky finger. It is found on both the left and right hands, between the base of the pinky finger and the wrist.

Corresponding meridian:

Small Intestine

Why we use it:

Releases feeling stuck and promotes ease in moving forward, letting go, healing from grief, and becoming happy in the present moment.

Tips for Tapping:

You can tap on either hand, using the opposite hand to do the tapping. Try using several fingers from the opposite hand to tap on this point. I personally like to use all four fingers to tap along the length of the side of my hand to stimulate the Side of the Hand point.

2. Eyebrow (EB)

Location:

This point is where your hair begins on the inner part of your eyebrow, right on the bone there. It is found on both sides of the body, on both the left and the right brow bone.

Corresponding meridian:

Bladder

Why we use it:

Releases trauma, hurt, and sadness and promotes peace and emotional healing.

Tips for Tapping:

You can tap on both sides at once, pick just one side of the body, or alternate sides as you go along. Try using just a few fingers, like the index and middle fingers, to tap on this point.

3. Side of the Eye (SE)

Location:

From the Eyebrow point, follow that ridge of bone from your eyebrow down to the side of the eye to find this point. Note that the Side of the Eye point is not located in the indent that is your temple; you'll want to stay on top of the bone instead.

Corresponding meridian:

Gallbladder

Why we use it:

Releases resentment and anger and promotes clarity and compassion.

Tips for Tapping:

You can tap on both sides at once, pick just one side of the body, or alternate sides as you go along. Try using just a few fingers, like the index and middle fingers, to tap on this point.

4. Under the Eye (UE)

Location:

From the Side of the Eye Tapping point, follow that ridge of bone once again to come under your eye. This point is found directly under the eye, on either side of the body.

Corresponding meridian:

Stomach

Why we use it:

Releases fear and anxiety and promotes feelings of contentment, calmness, and safety.

Tips for Tapping:

You can tap on both sides at once, pick just one side of the body, or alternate sides as you go along. Try using just a few fingers, like the index and middle fingers, to tap on this point.

5. Under the Nose (UN)

Location:

This point is found in the space between your nose and upper lip.

Corresponding meridian:

Governing Vessel

Why we use it:

Releases shame and powerlessness and promotes self-acceptance, self-empowerment, and compassion for self and others.

Tips for Tapping:

As it is a small area, try using just a few fingers (like the index and middle fingers) to reach this point for Tapping.

6. Under the Mouth (UM)

Location:

Also called the chin point, this point is found in the crease between your chin and bottom lip.

Corresponding meridian:

Central

Why we use it:

Releases confusion and uncertainty and promotes clarity, certainty, confidence, and self-acceptance.

Tips for Tapping:

As it is a small area, try using just a few fingers (like the index and middle fingers) to reach this point for Tapping.

7. Collarbone (CB)

Location:

Starting from where your collarbones meet in the center (at the base of that U-shape), go down one inch and out one inch to either side to get to the Collarbone point. This Tapping point is found on both the left and right sides of the body.

Corresponding meridian:

Kidney

Why we use it:

Releases the feeling of being stuck, promotes ease in moving forward, and boosts confidence and clarity.

Tips for Tapping:

You can tap with a few fingers on either side of the body to stimulate this point. Alternatively, try taking your whole hand and tapping the entire hand across the place where a bowtie would lie. That allows you to easily stimulate this point on both sides at once without having to worry about the exact location of the point.

8. Under the Arm (UA)

Location:

This point is located on your side, about four inches (or one hand's width) below the armpit. That is about where a bra strap lies. It is found on both the left and right side of the body.

Corresponding meridian:

Spleen

Why we use it:

Releases guilt, worry, and obsessing and promotes clarity, confidence, relaxation, and compassion for self and others.

Tips for Tapping:

The easiest way to stimulate this point is to use all your fingers, or your whole hand, to tap on the side of the body under your arm.

9. Top of the Head (TH)

Location:

This point is right on the center of the top of your head, at the crown.

Corresponding meridian:

This isn't necessarily one particular point, but rather a collection of many meridian points. Along with being associated with several of the meridians, the Top of the Head point is also connected to the crown chakra.

Why we use it:

Opens the crown chakra and promotes spiritual connection, while anchoring in the new balance and alignment from the Tapping round that has just been completed.

Tips for Tapping:

Simply tap your hand or your fingertips at the very top of your head to stimulate this Tapping point.

Note:

The emotional and psychological benefits associated with each Tapping point are rooted in traditional Chinese medicine and acupuncture theory, which holds that energy (or "qi") flows through the body along pathways called meridians. Each meridian corresponds to specific organs and is believed to influence particular emotional states. While these associations come from thousands of years of practice and observation in traditional Chinese medicine, they reflect traditional wisdom rather than modern scientific conclusions. We find this framework fascinating and wanted to share it above to provide context for the Tapping points.

Appendix B

Frequently Asked Questions

Getting Started

How hard do I tap?

Think Goldilocks here—not too hard, not too soft, just right. About the same pressure you'd use to drum your fingers on a table when you're thinking. You want to feel it, but it should never be uncomfortable. Your body will tell you what feels good.

Which side of my body should I tap on?

Either side works! The meridian points run down both sides of your body, so tap on whichever side feels more natural. If you can, tap on both sides at once, or feel free to switch it up.

What if I can't remember all the points? What if I mess it up?

Even if you only remember three points and tap those over and over, you'll still get benefits. Think of it like exercise—doing three push-ups is better than zero push-ups. The more accurately you can pinpoint the spots, the better (try not to tap in the middle of your forehead if you can!), but just do your best. Check out the reference guide on page 295 to dial in your practice.

Do I have to say the words out loud or can I think them?

Both work! Saying them out loud can be more powerful because we tend to be more engaged when speaking, but thinking the words absolutely counts. If you're in a public place or just prefer privacy, feel free to repeat in your mind instead of out loud.

What if the words don't resonate or feel true for me?

Change them! The scripts in this book and in our guided meditations are starting points, not scripture. The magic isn't in specific words—it's in acknowledging what's true for you while you tap. Make it yours.

The Experience

Is it normal to yawn/cry/feel tingling/get sleepy while Tapping?

Totally normal! These are actually great signs that energy is moving and your nervous system is shifting. Yawning is one of the most common—it's your body's way of releasing. Tears, tingling, sighing, even burping . . . all normal. Your body is letting go of stored stress. Celebrate these weird little moments—they mean it's working.

Why do I sometimes feel worse before I feel better?

Because you're actually processing things instead of avoiding them or pushing them down. It's like cleaning out a closet—things get messier before they get more organized. Stick with it—the relief on the other side is worth it.

How long before I see results?

Some people feel different after one round of tapping. Others need a few sessions or weeks of regular practice. It's like asking, "How long before I get fit?"—it depends on where you're starting and what you're working on. Trust that every round of Tapping is doing something, even if you can't feel it yet. The shifts often sneak up on you.

What if nothing happens when I tap?

Sometimes change is subtle—like realizing you slept better or didn't snap at your kids. If you truly feel nothing after consistent practice, you might be Tapping on surface stuff while the real issue hides underneath. Try getting more specific to dig deeper.

Can Tapping bring up old memories or emotions?

Yes, and that's actually a good thing (though it might not feel like it in the moment). Your brain stores everything, and Tapping can unlock filed-away experiences that still affect you. If something intense surfaces, keep tapping through it. This is all part of the rewiring process.

Why do I resist tapping even though I know it helps?

Because your brain loves familiar suffering more than unfamiliar peace. Seriously. That resistance is your nervous system saying, "Change is scary! Stick with what we know!" If this happens for you, try Tapping on the resistance itself in order to release it.

Practical Application

When is the best time to tap?

Whenever you'll actually do it. Morning Tapping sets a calm tone for your day. Evening Tapping helps you decompress. But the best time? Whenever you need it. Mind racing, can't sleep, or notice yourself spiraling? Don't wait for the "perfect" time—tap when you need it.

How often should I tap?

There's no one-size-fits-all answer to how often you should tap. You can tap several times per day, or once a week—whatever works for you! We do recommend committing to a daily practice so that you can get in the habit of using this tool regularly.

Listening to your body is a great way to know how much Tapping is right for you. If you are feeling rested and calm, then great! Keep Tapping! But if you are feeling like your body is exhausted and worn out and you could use a break, then it might be time to rest up. The emotional shifts can be a lot to process, so stay hydrated, rest, and practice self-care.

Can children use Tapping?

Tapping is an excellent tool for kids! It is super simple to do, and kids tend to pick it up really quickly! Tapping has been shown to have numerous benefits for children, including: reducing anxiety, boosting self-confidence, improving focus and concentration, enhancing academic performance, sleeping better, and more. Schools and parents nationwide are using this proven technique to help kids overcome stress and become more calm and confident. We have an entire section in our Tapping Solution App dedicated to content for kids. We even have video sessions for kids, led by other kids, to make the process even more fun, easy, and effective.

How do I know if I need professional help?

If you're experiencing symptoms of a mental or physical health condition, always consult with a medical professional for guidance. Tapping is powerful, but it's not a replacement for therapy or medical care when you really need it. Many therapists now incorporate Tapping into their practice—best of both worlds. Working with a Tapping practitioner can be particularly helpful if you are working with difficult memories, trauma, or intense symptoms.

What is The Tapping Solution App?

The Tapping Solution App is an all-inclusive resource to help you integrate Tapping into your daily life. In The Tapping Solution App, we've carefully crafted over 1,000 sessions to guide you through the Tapping process. Our Tapping meditations range from just two minutes to longer, more in-depth meditations. We even have video sessions so you can follow along in real time as we tap together. In addition to Tapping sessions, the app also includes features like Tapping Challenges, Audiobooks, Daily Inspiration audios, and a universe of other healing modalities (like affirmations, guided imagery, Sleep Journeys, walking meditations, and more!).

Visit www.thetappingsolution.com/rewired to learn more.

The Skeptic's Corner

How can something so simple actually work?

Tapping sends calming signals through multiple channels simultaneously: acupressure points, bilateral stimulation, focused attention, and verbal processing. So while it may seem like it at first glance, it's not really that simple—it's a multimodal intervention packaged in a basic technique. Your nervous system doesn't need something complicated to rewire old patterns—it just needs the right approach.

Is this just the placebo effect?

We have brain scans, cortisol tests, genetic expression analysis, and 300-plus other studies showing real biological changes. And several studies have shown that the physical act of tapping on these specific points is an active ingredient in the Tapping process. Sure, believing it helps probably enhances the effects, but Tapping creates measurable shifts whether you believe in it or not.

Why haven't I heard about this from my doctor or therapist?

Mainstream systems sometimes take a while to catch up with what's making a difference. It took decades for meditation and acupuncture to go mainstream, and they still aren't universally accepted. We're excited to see that many doctors, therapists, hospitals, clinics, coaches, and other practitioners are already using Tapping, but systemic change takes time.

Appendix C

Deep-Dive Scientific Evidence for Fellow Nerds

If you're the type who reads scientific papers for fun and loves getting into the weeds of research (we see you!), this section is for you. While the main book focuses on the practical side of Tapping, here we'll dive a bit deeper into the research that backs it up.

When I first started teaching Tapping 20 years ago, we had passionate testimonials but limited hard science. Today? We're swimming in gold-standard research that would make any skeptic pause. What you're about to read represents thousands of hours of rigorous scientific investigation across multiple continents, all asking the same question: Does this weird face-tapping thing actually work? Spoiler alert: It really, really does.

Get ready for effect sizes, cortisol measurements, brain scans, and all the nerdy goodness that shows why this simple technique creates such profound changes.

The Big Picture: Over 300 Studies and Counting

As of 2025, over 300 studies on EFT Tapping have been published, including:

- 103 Randomized Controlled Trials (RCTs)—the gold standard of research
- 19 meta-analyses and systematic reviews
- 95 pre-post outcome studies
- Studies from investigators in 12-plus countries

This breadth of research matters because it shows Tapping works across cultures, conditions, and contexts. When something helps veterans in the US, genocide survivors in Rwanda, and nursing students in Turkey, you know you're dealing with a universal human response, not a cultural quirk.

This isn't some fringe technique anymore; it's been put through the scientific wringer and come out stronger.

Your Stress Hormones on Tapping: The Cortisol Studies

Let's start with the hormone that makes you feel wired and tired at the same time: cortisol. This is commonly referred to as the stress hormone.

Tapping has been shown repeatedly to decrease cortisol levels, and fast.

This "stress hormone" isn't just about feeling stressed; it affects everything from your immune system to your ability to form memories. Chronically elevated cortisol is linked to depression, anxiety, weight gain, heart disease, and even shrinking of brain regions involved in memory. So when we can measurably reduce cortisol, we're not just helping you feel better—we're profoundly influencing your long-term health and your quality of life.

The Landmark Study[14]

- 83 participants randomized to: EFT Tapping, supportive talk therapy, or rest
- After just *one hour*:
    - EFT group: 24% cortisol drop
    - Supportive talk therapy: 14% drop
    - Rest: 14% drop
- Translation: Tapping reduced stress hormones 10% more than standard treatment

The Mind-Blowing Replication Study[15]

- In 2020, a new set of researchers set out to replicate those results
- They found even bigger results: a 43% cortisol reduction in cortisol with an hour of EFT Tapping
- That translates to cutting your stress hormone nearly in *half* in one session
- Control group showed only a 20% reduction

The Workshop Study[16]

- 203 participants at a four-day EFT workshop
- Results: 37% decrease in resting cortisol
- Bonus: Benefits sustained at one-year follow-up
- Extra bonus: 113% increase in an immune marker (secretory IgA, or SIgA), suggesting enhanced immune function

What Your Brain Looks Like on Tapping: Neuroimaging Studies

Brain imaging changed everything for Tapping research. Suddenly, we could *see* the changes happening in real time. It's one thing to say, "I feel better," and it's another to show the brain actually responding differently when Tapping comes into play.

The Food Craving fMRI Study[17]

- 15 overweight adults with intense food cravings
- Performed brain scans while looking at pictures of junk food before they tried EFT Tapping for four weeks
- After four weeks of EFT:
    - 18% reduction in cravings (vs. 5% for controls)
    - Brain scans showed decreased activation in reward centers related to cravings
- Translation: The "I *need* that" part of the brain calmed down, and no longer lit up when looking at tempting foods

The Chronic Pain fMRI Study[18]

- Chronic pain sufferers received EFT treatment, with fMRI studies done before and after the Tapping
- Brain scans revealed decreased connectivity in pain modulation and catastrophizing regions

- Translation: Tapping doesn't just help you cope with pain; it changes how your brain processes pain signals
- Results across the board:
    - Pain severity: ↓21%
    - Pain interference: ↓26%
    - Somatic symptoms: ↓28%
    - Depression: ↓13%
    - Anxiety: ↓37%
    - Quality of life: ↑7%
    - Happiness: ↑17%
    - Life satisfaction: ↑9%

EEG Brain Wave Studies[19]

- Multiple studies show EFT creates brain wave patterns similar to deep meditation and "flow" states
- Tapping linked to suppression of high-frequency beta waves (the anxiety waves) and increase in alpha/theta waves (the relaxed, flow-state waves)
- Findings suggest EFT Tapping shifts the brain from stressed and aroused to relaxed and receptive

PTSD and Trauma: Where EFT Really Shines

If there's one area where Tapping has completely revolutionized treatment, it's trauma. Traditional trauma therapy often takes years and can be incredibly difficult. The studies below show something remarkable: Tapping allows people to process trauma without drowning in it, and find relief fast. Veterans who've carried combat trauma for 40 years find peace. Genocide survivors reclaim their lives. The research doesn't just show marginal improvements—it shows complete transformations. And those transformations are happening faster than anyone thought possible.

The evidence here is so strong, it's changing how we think about trauma treatment.

Veterans Study (Church et al. 2013)[20]

- Veterans who'd suffered for *decades*
- After just six one-hour EFT Tapping sessions:
  - 90% of the EFT group no longer met PTSD criteria
  - Control group: Only 4% improvement
  - Results showed sustained improvements over long-term follow-ups

Rwanda Genocide Survivors (Sakai et al. 2010)[21]

- 50 orphaned teenagers with severe PTSD
- After *one* Thought Field Therapy session (the precursor to EFT Tapping):
  - 100% of group meeting PTSD criteria → 6% meeting PTSD criteria (based on caregiver reports)
  - When looking at self-reports of PTSD symptoms, the numbers went from 72% → 18%
- One year later, all the improvements held strong

Recent Meta-Analysis[22]

- Meta analysis including 13 studies and 621 patients
- Concluded that EFT effectively treats PTSD and comorbid symptoms including anxiety and depression when compared to control groups
- Effect size: -2.1 (that's *huge* in psychology terms)
- Benefits sustained three months after Tapping treatment

If Tapping can help these groups—genocide survivors, veterans, etc., imagine what it could do for others dealing with trauma?

Anxiety: Rapid Relief Backed by Data

Anxiety is your brain's smoke alarm going off when there's no fire. Traditional treatments try to teach you to live with the alarm, to breathe through it, to understand why it's ringing. Tapping does something different by recalibrating the alarm system itself. The studies below show that in as little as one session, people experience significant drops in anxiety that last. Not temporary relief that fades by tomorrow, but genuine rewiring of the anxiety response. For the millions of us lying awake at 3 A.M. with racing thoughts, these studies offer more than hope; they offer a proven path to greater ease.

Meta-Analysis[23]

- Meta-analysis including 14 studies and 658 participants
- Found that EFT Tapping produced a significant reduction in anxiety
- Effect size for Tapping: $d = 1.23$ (considered a very large effect)
- Many studies used just one to four sessions, much shorter than other standard anxiety treatments like therapy

Real-World Example: Test Anxiety[24]

- 80 nursing students in Turkey
- Three EFT sessions done in a group setting reduced test anxiety and helped them cope better with other stressors

Depression: Surprising Strength

Traditional treatments often help with depression, but they can take months to work and come with challenging side effects. The studies below reveal something extraordinary: Tapping consistently shows effect sizes two to four times larger than conventional treatments. People who've been trapped in darkness for decades suddenly find windows opening. Not because they're forcing happiness, but because Tapping addresses depression at its core.

Meta-Analysis[25]

- 18 studies analyzed

- Results suggested that EFT alleviates depressive symptoms
- Overall effect size: d = 1.27 (considered a very large effect size, bigger than most traditional treatments show)
- For context: Antidepressants typically showed = 0.3–0.5

Recent Review [26]

- Mean symptom reduction: 41%
- That's cutting depression symptoms nearly in half

Stress, Distress, and Physiological Outcomes

Stress isn't just in your head; it's in every cell of your body. Chronic stress disrupts everything from your heart rate to your immune system, from your blood pressure to your cellular aging. It's like running your car engine with "check engine" on 24/7—eventually, everything starts breaking down.

The studies in this section show that Tapping doesn't just help you feel calmer, but it also creates measurable improvements in the biological markers that determine how long and how well you'll live. We're talking about changes you can measure with a blood test, a blood pressure cuff, and immune system markers.

The Workshop Study Strikes Again[27]

- Heart rate: ↓8%
- Blood pressure: ↓6–8%
- Immune marker: ↑113%

Church[28]

- Found that one EFT Tapping session led to a 50% reduction in total symptom distress (versus little change in controls)
- Documented improvements across anxiety, depression, and other stress-related symptoms

Real-World Evidence: 32 Million Sessions Can't Be Wrong

Laboratory studies are crucial, but what really matters is: Does this work in real life? When people are stressed about bills, fighting with their spouse, or panicking at 2 A.M.? The data from The Tapping Solution App represents the largest real-world study of any mind-body technique ever conducted. These aren't paid research subjects in controlled conditions; they're people like you, tapping in their cars, their bedrooms, their office bathrooms. And the results are even more impressive than the lab studies, showing that Tapping works wherever you are, whatever you're facing.

The Tapping Solution App Study[29]

- 380,000-plus Tapping sessions analyzed
- 96,000 users over one year
- Average anxiety reduction per session: 29.1%
- Average stress reduction: 30.8%
- All results highly significant ($p < .001$)

Sessions in the App Have Now Been Played over 32 Million Times

Top-performing sessions:

- "Releasing Anxiety": 1.7 million plays, average approximately 40% reduction
- "Quiet My Racing Mind": 1 million plays, average approximately 47% reduction
- "You Are Enough": 615,000 plays, average approximately 48% reduction

The Safety Profile: Basically Zero Risk

Across all these studies:

- No significant adverse events reported
- No negative side effects
- Often produces "side benefits" (better sleep, improved mood)
- Safe for children, elderly, and other sensitive groups

The Mechanisms: How Does Tapping Actually Work?

For years, critics dismissed Tapping because we couldn't explain exactly *how* it worked. Now we know more and more by the year. The research reveals that Tapping orchestrates changes across multiple body systems simultaneously. It's not just one mechanism—it's a symphony of healing responses all triggered by this simple technique:

1. **HPA Axis Regulation:** Calms your stress response system
2. **Limbic System Deactivation:** Turns down your brain's alarm system
3. **Memory Reconsolidation:** Updates traumatic memories with calm
4. **Vagal Tone Enhancement:** Activates your rest-and-digest system
5. **Gene Expression Changes:** Has even been shown to affect how your genes work[30]

What This Means for You

If you've made it this far into the research rabbit hole, here's the bottom line: Tapping isn't just "woo-woo"—it's one of the most studied mind-body techniques out there. The evidence shows it can create rapid, lasting changes in your brain, body, and emotional state.

Whether you're dealing with that 3 A.M. anxiety spiral, chronic pain, trauma from decades ago, or just everyday stress, there's solid science showing Tapping can help. And unlike many interventions, it's free, has no side effects, and you can do it anywhere.

Remember: You don't need to understand all the science to benefit from Tapping. But for those of us who love knowing the "why" behind the "how," isn't it amazing that something so simple is backed by so much evidence?

Now go forth and tap! Science has your back.

Want Even More Research?

For more studies and additional research, visit www.thetappingsolution.com/rewired or scan the QR code.

Appendix D

Tapping for Every Area of Life

You've learned the foundation. You've tapped through the core challenges covered in this book. Now here's what's important to understand: Tapping works on way more than what we covered in these pages.

This appendix lists categories and sessions from The Tapping Solution App to show you the wide range of specific issues and areas that Tapping can work on. We want you to see the breadth of just how much Tapping can help with. Scan through and notice which topics make you think, "Wait, I didn't know Tapping could help with *that*."

If any of these topics speak to you, go explore them in the app. Some sessions are free, some are available with a paid membership.

Learn more at www.thetappingsolution.com/rewired or download The Tapping Solution App.

Aging Mindfully

As we age, our relationship with our body and identity shifts. Tapping helps release fears about aging, body changes, and loss of vitality while cultivating acceptance and discovering new possibilities. It rewires limiting beliefs about what's possible "at your age" and helps you embrace this phase with grace.

Cancer Support

A cancer diagnosis triggers the nervous system into high alert. Tapping provides gentle support through treatment, helping manage fear, nausea, and exhaustion. Tapping gives you a tool to actively participate in your healing, find clarity, and navigate the journey with greater ease.

Caregiver Support

Caring for others while running on high alert creates dangerous depletion. Tapping helps caregivers release guilt about self-care, process daily stress, and restore their own energy reserves.

CBT and Tapping: The Power of Combined Therapies

Tapping is ideal for enhancing CBT work. This powerful combination addresses both the mental understanding and the body's stress response, creating faster, more lasting change. Think sessions like Break Free from Unhelpful Habits, Change Unhelpful Thought Pattern, Transform Limiting Beliefs, and Understand and Release Emotions.

Calm Your Mind

Tapping interrupts the circuits of racing thoughts, mental loops, and overthinking and creates space between you and your thoughts. Think Tapping sessions particularly designed for:

- Worry
- Racing Thoughts
- Assuming the Worst
- Overthinking
- Memories That Keep Replaying
- Thoughts About Something *You* Did or Said
- Thoughts About Something Someone *Else* Did or Said

Chakra Balancing

Whether you view chakras as energy centers or metaphors for different life areas, Tapping combines ancient wisdom with modern neuroscience to address blockages, restore flow, and help you tune in to different themes in your life: from safety and grounding to intuition and connection.

Daily Tapping Tune-ups

Your nervous system needs daily maintenance just like your teeth need brushing. Daily tune-ups keep your system regulated, preventing stress buildup and maintaining the calm baseline you've worked to create.

Emotional Freedom

Emotions are meant to flow through you, not get stuck inside. Tapping helps release trapped emotions while building your capacity to feel without drowning. Whether you're dealing with anxiety, depression, grief, or just feeling "blah," Tapping is incredibly powerful for restoring emotional balance and freedom.

Just a few of the specific emotions we cover in the app:

- Anger
- Anxiety
- Betrayal
- Disappointment
- Grief
- Grief over the loss of a pet
- Jealousy
- Loneliness
- Pain of rejection
- Regret
- Resentment
- Self-doubt
- Shame
- Winter blues

Fears and Phobias

Fears and phobias hijack your nervous system, causing you to avoid experiences that could enrich your life. Tapping helps rewire your brain's threat assessment, helping you distinguish between real danger and false alarms. Try it to transform paralyzing fear into manageable concern, reclaiming activities and experiences you've been avoiding.

Some of the fears and phobias that we include in this category:

- Fear of Dogs
- Fear of Driving
- Fear of Flying
- Fear of Heights
- Fear of Needles
- Fear of Public Speaking
- Fear of Small Spaces (Claustrophobia)
- Fear of Snakes
- Fear of Spiders
- Fear of the Dentist
- Fear of the Doctor
- Fear of Throwing Up
- Social Anxiety

Inner Child Healing

Many of our deepest patterns formed in childhood when we didn't have the resources to process big experiences. Tapping helps you reconnect with and reparent your inner child, giving them the safety, validation, and love they needed then. This healing ripples forward, transforming how you show up today.

I'm Stressed About . . .

Life throws countless stressors our way—from family dynamics to financial pressure to global uncertainty. Targeted Tapping sessions for specific stress triggers can help us move from Reactive Loops to responsive calm.

We have sessions for all of the following:

- I'm Stressed About Change
- I'm Stressed About My Children
- I'm Stressed About My Family
- I'm Stressed About My Health
- I'm Stressed About Money
- I'm Stressed About My Spouse
- I'm Stressed About My Taxes
- I'm Stressed About My Weight
- I'm Stressed About Politics
- I'm Stressed About Uncertainty
- I'm Stressed About Work
- I'm Stressed About the World

Instant and Micro Boosts (three to eight minutes)

Like little pep talks, shorter Tapping sessions can be incredibly helpful for giving you a boost of energy, happiness, healing, and more! Targeting a specific topic can help to uplift your mind, body, and day. Think topics like courage, energy, focus, hope, patience, peace, safety, inner strength, and joy.

There are also short Tapping sessions to help you prepare for specific situations and events, such as:

- Pre-Athletic Event Micro Boost
- Pre-Date Micro Boost
- Pre–Important Discussion Micro Boost
- Pre-Interview Micro Boost
- Pre–Meeting New People Micro Boost
- Pre-Performance Micro Boost
- Pre-Presentation Micro Boost
- Pre-Social Activity Micro Boost
- Pre-Test Micro Boost

Motivate Me To . . .

Whether you are trying to work, write, exercise, clear clutter, eat better, or make a decision, Tapping can help you release resistance to taking action on what you need to, so you can feel focused and empowered.

Pain Relief

There are many ways that the brain and body can create, increase, and prolong pain. Tapping has been shown to reduce and even eliminate physical pain—as well as help with the emotional distress caused by pain and a diagnosis.

The app offers specific sessions for all sorts of pain, including:

- Arthritis pain
- Back pain
- Chronic pain
- Endometriosis pain
- Headache
- Intestinal pain
- Knee pain
- Neck pain
- Neuropathic pain
- Pelvis pain
- Postoperative pain
- Sciatic Pain
- Sinus Pain
- Stomach pain
- Sore throat

Performance Support

Whether you're at an open mic night or on Broadway, Tapping can help you channel nervous energy into powerful presence, so you can show up as your best self.

Relationships

Tapping can help you stay regulated during conflicts, release old patterns, and create healthier dynamics. Because changing your internal wiring changes how you show up with others.

Try Tapping sessions on everything from Breakup Support and Dating Support to Clearing Negative Energy Picked Up from Others and Preparing for a Difficult Conversation at Work.

Sleep Support

Sleep struggles aren't just about being tired. They're your nervous system stuck in "danger" mode when it should switch to "safe." Tapping can help reset your sleep circuitry, quiet racing thoughts, and train your body to welcome rest.

Try Tapping sessions to help you fall asleep faster, fall back asleep, quiet your racing mind, or get more deep sleep.

Sports Performance

Elite athletes know that mental game determines physical performance. From speeding up recovery to getting into the flow state to performing under pressure, Tapping can help with many aspects of athletics.

Support Your Body

Your body's symptoms often reflect nervous system dysregulation. While not a replacement for medical care, Tapping can help calm the body's responses, address underlying stress patterns, address physical symptoms, and help you feel empowered as you navigate health challenges big or small.

This category covers a wide range of health concerns, such as:

- Allergies
- Asthma
- Autoimmune Conditions
- Cancer
- Cholesterol
- Chronic Lyme Disease
- Cigarette Cravings and Quitting Smoking
- Diabetes
- Dizziness and Vertigo
- Eczema
- Glaucoma
- Gut Issues
- Hair Loss
- Headaches
- Heart Health
- Hormone Health
- IBS
- Indigestion, Acid Reflux, and More
- Jaw Health/TMJ
- Kidney Health
- Liver Health
- Lung Issues
- MCAS
- Misophonia
- Opioid Detox
- Plantar Fasciitis

- Psoriasis
- Restless Legs Syndrome
- Skin Health
- Thyroid Health
- Tinnitus
- Ulcers

You can also find support for specific symptoms, such as:

- Constipation
- Fatigue
- Fever
- Headache
- Jet Lag
- Nasal Congestion
- Nausea
- Sore Throat

Tapping for Kids

Children's nervous systems are still developing, making them especially responsive to Tapping. Kid-friendly Tapping sessions help young ones manage big emotions, sleep better, and build resilience. Teaching kids to tap gives them a superpower for life.

Your kids can tap along to sessions on issues like stress, test anxiety, frustration with a sibling, bad dreams, self-doubt, jealousy, and peer pressure, plus they can do uplifting sessions to boost confidence, calm, gratitude, joy, and creativity.

Tapping and Breathwork Collection

Combining Tapping with specific breathing patterns amplifies both practices. Breathwork regulates your nervous system while Tapping rewires it; together they create profound shifts in minutes. Perfect for anxiety, focus, or deep relaxation.

Trauma Support

Trauma lives in the body, not just the mind. Tapping can be a powerful tool to help you safely process and release pain from the past, so you can restore safety, build resilience, and reclaim the parts of yourself that went into hiding.

Turn Your Day Around

Bad days happen, but they don't have to stay bad. Tapping is the perfect tool to interrupt downward spirals and pivot you toward greater ease. Whether it's morning stress or afternoon overwhelm, you can use Tapping to reset your nervous system and reclaim your day.

Some user favorite Tapping meditations include:

- Afternoon Reset
- Change a Bad Day
- Create a Great Day
- Evening Stress Relief
- Morning Stress Relief
- Quieting the Critical Voice
- Release Overwhelm
- Stop a Panic Attack

Vagus Nerve Toning

Your vagus nerve is the master switch between stress and calm. Tapping to target vagal tone can be effective in enhancing your body's ability to self-regulate. Think of it as strength training for your nervous system's peace response.

Wealth and Abundance

If you are looking for more abundance to flow into your life, but still holding on to old thought patterns of struggle and lack, Tapping can help. Try Tapping to release any mental blocks, calm the panic that prevents clear financial thinking, and open yourself up to allow new and fresh opportunities to enter your life.

Weight Loss and Body Confidence

Tapping addresses the underlying emotions driving food behaviors while building genuine body acceptance, so you can heal your relationship with food, your body, and your sense of confidence all simultaneously.

From Cravings Buster meditations to sessions to help you direct more love and compassion toward your body, this category helps from all angles.

Women's Health

Women face unique challenges through fertility, pregnancy, menstruation, and menopause. Tapping to calm the nervous system can help address any physical symptoms while also supporting the emotional journey.

This category includes our collections for:

- Early Motherhood Support
- Fertility and IVF Support
- Menopause Support
- Menstrual Cycle Support
- Pregnancy Support
- And more

Workplace Wellness

Work stress doesn't have to follow you home. Tapping is quite effective in helping you stay regulated during difficult meetings, recover from setbacks, and maintain confidence as you navigate your career. From Clear and Focused for Work to Rebound from Losing a Deal, this category covers a wide range of workplace challenges and needs.

You Are Enough

At the core of most struggles is the belief that we're not enough. Tapping helps rewire this fundamental pattern, building genuine self-worth from the inside out. And when you know you're enough, everything else shifts.

The Tapping Solution Foundation

Through our Foundation, we bring free Tapping resources to communities in crisis and to groups who can use extra support. These specialized sessions support those on the frontlines of trauma and service, helping healers stay regulated so they can continue their vital work.

We have specialized collections for Events and Global Support, First Responders, Teachers, Military and Veterans, and Healthcare Providers.

Endnotes

1. Dawson Church, Garret Yount, and Audrey Brooks, "The Effect of Emotional Freedom Techniques on Stress Biochemistry: A Randomized Controlled Trial," *Journal of Nervous and Mental Disease* 200, no.10 (2012): 891–96, https://doi.org/10.1097/NMD.0b013e31826b9fc1; and Peta Stapleton et al., "Reexamining the Effect of Emotional Freedom Techniques on Stress Biochemistry: A Randomized Controlled Trial," *Psychological Trauma: Theory, Research, Practice, and Policy* 12, no. 8 (2020): 869–77, https://doi.org/10.1037/tra0000563.

2. Marjorie E. Maharaj, "Differential Gene Expression After Emotional Freedom Techniques (EFT) Treatment: A Novel Pilot Protocol for Salivary mRNA Assessment," *Energy Psychology Journal: Theory, Research & Treatment* 8, no. 1 (2016): 12–25, https://energypsychologyjournal.org/differential-gene-expression-emotional-freedom-techniques-eft-treatment-novel-pilot-protocol-salivary-mrna-assessment/.

3. Donna Bach et al., "Clinical EFT (Emotional Freedom Techniques) Improves Multiple Physiological Markers of Health," *Journal of Evidence-Based Integrative Medicine* 24 (2019): 1–12, https://doi.org/10.1177/2515690X18823691.

4. Peta Stapleton et al., "Neural Changes After Emotional Freedom Techniques Treatment for Chronic Pain," *Complementary Therapies in Clinical Practice* 49 (2022): 101653. https://doi.org/10.1016/j.ctcp.2022.101653; and Peta Stapleton et al., "An Initial Investigation of Neural Changes in Overweight Adults with Food Cravings After Emotional Freedom Techniques," *OBM Integrative and Complementary Medicine* 4, no. 1 (2019): 1–10, https://doi.org/10.21926/obm.icm.1901010.

5. Dawson Church et al., "Clinical EFT as an Evidence-Based Practice for the Treatment of Psychological and Physiological Conditions: A Systematic Review," *Frontiers in Psychology* 13 (2022): 951451, https://doi.org/10.3389/fpsyg.2022.951451.

6. Dawson Church et al., "Psychological Trauma Symptom Improvement in Veterans Using Emotional Freedom Techniques: A Randomized Controlled Trial," *Journal of Nervous and Mental Disease* 201, no. 2 (2013): 153–60, https://doi.org/10.1097/NMD.0b013e31827f6351.

7. Peta Stapleton, "Reexamining the Effect of Emotional Freedom Techniques on Stress Biochemistry," 869–77.

8. Morgan Clond, "Emotional Freedom Techniques for Anxiety: A Systematic Review with Meta-Analysis," *Journal of Nervous and Mental Disease* 204, no. 5 (2016): 388–95, https://doi.org/10.1097/NMD.0000000000000483.

9. Ji-Woo Seok and Jaeuk U. Kim, "The Effectiveness of Emotional Freedom Techniques for Depressive Symptoms: A Meta-Analysis," *Journal of Clinical Medicine* 13, no. 21 (2024): 6481, https://doi.org/10.3390/jcm13216481.

10. Daniela Schiller, "Unmaking Painful Memories," interview on *Road to Resilience* podcast, Mount Sinai, published July 15, 2020, https://www.mountsinai.org/about/newsroom/podcasts/road-resilience/archive/unmaking-painful-memories.

11. Dina Wittfoth et al., "Bifocal Emotion Regulation Through Acupoint Tapping in Fear of Flying," *Neuroimage: Clinical* 34 (2022): 102996, https://www.sciencedirect.com/science/article/pii/S2213158222000614.

12. A. Harvey Baker and Linda S. Siegel, "Emotional Freedom Techniques (EFT) Reduces Intense Fears: A Partial Replication and Extension of Wells, Polglase, Andrews, Carrington, & Baker (2003)," *Energy Psychology Journal: Theory, Research & Treatment* 2, no. 2 (2010): 13–30; and Steve Wells et al., "Evaluation of a Meridian-Based Intervention, Emotional Freedom Techniques (EFT), for Reducing Specific Phobias of Small Animals," *Journal of Clinical Psychol*ogy 59, no. 9 (2003): 943–66.

13. Caroline E. Sakai, Suzanne M. Connolly, and Paul Oas, "Treatment of PTSD in Rwandan Child Genocide Survivors Using Thought Field Therapy," *International Journal of Emergency Mental Health* 12, no. 1 (2010): 41–49, https://www.academia.edu/download/57257152/Sakai-Connolly-Oastudy.pdf.

14. Church, "The Effect of Emotional Freedom Techniques on Stress Biochemistry," 891–96.

15. Stapleton, "Reexamining the Effect of Emotional Freedom Techniques on Stress Biochemistry," 869–77.

16. Bach, "Clinical EFT (Emotional Freedom Techniques) Improves Multiple Physiological Markers of Health," 1–12.

17. Stapleton, "An Initial Investigation of Neural Changes in Overweight Adults," 1–10.

18. Stapleton, "Neural Changes After Emotional Freedom Techniques," 101653.

19. Judith Pennington, Debbie Sabot, and Dawson Church, "EcoMeditation and Emotional Freedom Techniques (EFT) Produce Elevated Brain-Wave Patterns and States of Consciousness," *Energy Psychology: Theory, Research & Treatment* 11, no. 1 (2019): 13–22, https://doi.org/10.9769/EPJ.2019.11.1.JP.

20. Church, "Psychological Trauma Symptom Improvement in Veterans," 153–60.

21. Sakai, "Treatment of PTSD in Rwandan Child Genocide Survivors," 41–49.

22. Wan-Ting Chen et al., "Effectiveness of Emotional Freedom Techniques in Alleviating Symptoms Associated with Posttraumatic Stress Disorder: A Systematic Review and Meta-Analysis," *European Archives of Psychiatry and Clinical Neuroscience* (2025), https://doi.org/10.1007/s00406-025-02000-4.

23. Clond, "Emotional Freedom Techniques for Anxiety," 388–95.

24. Pinar Irmak Vural, Gülşah Körpe, and Demet Inangil, "Emotional Freedom Techniques (EFT) to Reduce Exam Anxiety in Turkish Nursing Students," *European Journal of Integrative Medicine* 32 (2019): 101002, https://doi.org/10.1016/j.eujim.2019.101002.

25. Jerrod A. Nelms and Liana Castel, "A Systematic Review and Meta-Analysis of Randomized and Nonrandomized Trials of Clinical Emotional Freedom Techniques (EFT) for the Treatment of Depression," *Explore* 12, no 6 (2016): 416–26, https://doi.org/10.1016/j.explore.2016.08.001.

26. Seok, "The Effectiveness of Emotional Freedom Techniques for Depressive Symptoms," 6481.
27. Bach, "Clinical EFT (Emotional Freedom Techniques) Improves Multiple Physiological Markers of Health," 1–12.
28. Church, "The Effect of Emotional Freedom Techniques on Stress Biochemistry," 891–96.
29. Dawson Church, Peta Stapleton, and Debbie Sabot, "App-Based Delivery of Clinical Emotional Freedom Techniques: Cross-Sectional Study of App User Self-Ratings," *JMIR mHealth and uHealth* 8, no. 10 (2020): e18545, https://doi.org/10.2196/18545.
30. Maharaj, "Differential Gene Expression After Emotional Freedom Techniques (EFT) Treatment," 12–25.

Index

A

B

C

D

E

F

G

H

I

J

K

L

N

O

P

S

T

U

V

W

Acknowledgments

First, we want to thank our parents. Their courage to leave family behind and move to the United States opened doors we could never have imagined. Their love, resilience, and commitment to growth continue to inspire us every day.

We are deeply grateful to **Chelsea Clark**. Your editing, research, tireless work, and eagle eye for detail made this book what it is. Working with you is a true joy. Thank you **Julie Rosenberger**, for your hard work, patience, and talent to make everything look its best.

Thank you to **Reid Tracy**, our editor **Anne Barthel**, **Victoria Comella**, the entire team at **Hay House**, and the team at **Fortier** for your care, belief in this work, and dedication to bringing this book into the world.

To **The Tapping Solution team**, because of your heart-centered commitment, we are able to reach and support so many people. We are incredibly grateful to stand behind this work together.

And finally, thank you to everyone who shared their stories and to the countless readers who wrote with messages of support and breakthroughs. You are the heart of this book and why we do this work.

From Nick

Thank you to my wife, **Brenna**, whose love, patience, and belief in me make everything possible. I love you more every day. To **June** and **Ellis**—your silliness, your curiosity, and your giant hearts light up my life.

Thank you to **Tony Robbins**, who introduced me to Tapping 20 years ago and changed the course of my life. Your friendship and belief in this work over the years have meant more than you know. That you wrote the foreword to this book is a full-circle moment I never could have imagined.

From Jessica

Thank you to my husband, **Lucas**, who always helps me find my way out of my head and back into my heart. I love you. Thank you to **Enzo** and **Lucia**, who fill my life with so much love, joy, and meaning. And thank you to **Dee Mammano** and **Sarah Casey**, the godmothers, whose love for my children and unwavering support for me—through every step and misstep—means more than I can say.

From Alex

Thank you to my wife and partner in life, **Karen**—I love you more than you will ever know. Thank you to my three amazing kids, **Malakai**, **Lucas**, and **Olivia**. Being the best father I can be for you three has been and always will be my number one purpose and joy in life.

About the Authors

For more than fifteen years, siblings **Nick**, **Jessica**, and **Alex Ortner** have devoted their lives to a simple idea with world-shifting potential: that every person deserves tools to calm their mind, soothe their stress, and feel at home in their own body. What began as a small family project has grown into The Tapping Solution, a global movement that has helped millions reclaim their emotional well-being.

Together, they've created best-selling books, groundbreaking digital programs, and The Tapping Solution App, now the leading platform for EFT Tapping worldwide. With more than a thousand guided sessions played tens of millions of times, their work has brought evidence-based emotional relief into living rooms, classrooms, clinics, and communities around the globe.

Their impact extends beyond the screen. Through The Tapping Solution Foundation, the Ortners have brought Tapping to schools, disaster-relief zones, and underserved populations, offering practical tools in life's toughest moments.

The Ortners' mission is simple and profound: to make emotional relief accessible to all.

www.thetappingsolution.com

Hay House Titles of Related Interest

YOU CAN HEAL YOUR LIFE, the movie,
starring Louise Hay & Friends
(available as an online streaming video)
www.hayhouse.com/louise-movie

THE SHIFT, the movie,
starring Dr. Wayne W. Dyer
(available as an online streaming video)
www.hayhouse.com/the-shift-movie

***

BLISS BRAIN:
The Neuroscience of Remodeling Your Brain for Resilience, Creativity, and Joy,
by Dawson Church

DO THIS BEFORE BED:
Simple 5-Minute Practices That Will Change Your Life,
by Oliver Niño

LIMITLESS EXPANDED EDITION:
Upgrade Your Brain, Learn Anything Faster, and Unlock Your Exceptional Life,
by Jim Kwik

THE SCIENCE BEHIND TAPPING:
A Proven Stress Management Technique for the Mind and Body,
by Peta Stapleton, PhD

All of the above are available at your local bookstore,
or may be ordered by contacting Hay House (see next page).

***

We hope you enjoyed this Hay House book. If you'd like to receive our online catalog featuring additional information on Hay House books and products, or if you'd like to find out more about the Hay Foundation, please contact:

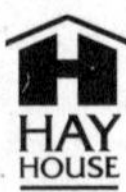

Hay House LLC, P.O. Box 5100, Carlsbad, CA 92018-5100
(760) 431-7695 or (800) 654-5126
www.hayhouse.com® • www.hayfoundation.org

Published in Australia by:
Hay House Australia Publishing Pty Ltd
18/36 Ralph St., Alexandria NSW 2015
Phone: +61 (02) 9669 4299
www.hayhouse.com.au

Published in the United Kingdom by:
Hay House UK Ltd
1st Floor, Crawford Corner,
91–93 Baker Street, London W1U 6QQ
Phone: +44 (0)20 3927 7290
www.hayhouse.co.uk

Published in India by:
Hay House Publishers (India) Pvt Ltd
Muskaan Complex, Plot No. 3,
B-2, Vasant Kunj, New Delhi 110 070
Phone: +91 11 41761620
www.hayhouse.co.in